# The
# Secret Lives
# of
# Fat People

# The
# Secret Lives
# of
# Fat People

## MILDRED KLINGMAN, M.S.W.

*Boston*

HOUGHTON MIFFLIN COMPANY

1981

*Library of Congress Cataloging
in Publication Data*
Klingman, Mildred.
The secret lives of fat people.
1. Obesity — Psychological aspects. I. Title.
[DNLM: 1. Obesity — Popular works. WD 212 K65g]
RC552.O25K56    616.3'98'0019    81–454
ISBN 0–395–31006–7            AACR1

Printed in the United States of America

P 10 9 8 7 6 5 4 3 2 1

The author is grateful to CBS News for permission to re-
print a segment from the *60 Minutes* program "Fat . . .
and Proud of It," which was originally broadcast on
December 10, 1978.

T*he Secret Lives of Fat People* is dedicated to the people who talked with me and to each other about being fat and to those who participated in the therapy groups. Their stories and feelings, painfully and honestly expressed, made it possible for me to write this book.

I have received much wonderful support and encouragement from the people around me, but am able to acknowledge only a few by name: My daughter, Lynnzee, my sons, David and Mark, Angela Scalpello, Nancy Weber, Chris Di Napoli, Mary Fenton, Mary O'Rourke, Mary DeWitt, Beverly D'Angelo, Robin Weiss.

I offer special thanks to Ellen Levine, my agent, to Anita McClellan, an extraordinary editor, to Judith Hennessee for her ability to disentangle confusion, and to John Gruber, for his insight and counsel.

# Contents

# Foreword

MOST AMERICANS think they are overweight. People who want to lose three or four pounds bemoan their fatness. On the other hand, many obese people believe they are "not that fat." Fat is a relative term, a state of mind. Whether they are among the mentally fat or the physically fat, fat people are unhappy about their weight.

In my work as a therapist, I began to see a pattern when fat people talked about how it feels to be fat. Emotionally, fat people have a lot in common. Being and feeling fat is the central fact of their lives. They virtually live to eat, funneling enormous amounts of energy into their eating habits and their feelings about food. Their thoughts circle endlessly around the last meal, the next meal, the way they look, how they can conceal their fat, how they can make others ignore it. Their greatest efforts go into adjusting their lives to their fatness.

Fat people talk about food as if it were a tranquilizer or a security blanket. They eat to avoid facing problems and refuse to take responsibility for their weight. Each of my fat clients developed a repertoire of deceptions, a string of secrets to hide the truth, to help them pretend their fat didn't exist. Food and fat and feelings became the building stones of a little walled city of which each fat person was the sole inhabitant, shut off from other people and from the lives they wanted to lead.

During group therapy sessions, my clients listened to their own self-defeating eating patterns being unraveled by others. As they became more aware of the real motivations behind their overeating, they began to understand why all their attempts to diet had failed, why they were still fat. They gained unexpected insights into their actions — actions that prevented them from losing weight. Something happened. The shock of recognition was strong enough to motivate some of them to begin to lose weight. To change their lives.

The experience of helping my clients was a source of deep personal gratification. It led me to write *The Secret Lives of Fat People* in the belief that looking at others in the book will motivate fat readers to lose weight. All the people I quote have created unnecessary unhappiness for themselves. It is my intention that these voices touch a nerve, set off a reaction that will help other people face their own truths. I hope the book will reveal why diets fail and, by showing how some fat people have lost weight and kept it off, help others become thin. Finally, it is my purpose to help fat people understand that by losing weight they are not depriving themselves but giving to themselves.

Being fat is not an incurable disease with occasional remissions during diets. Fat people don't have to be fat all their lives. The decision can be revoked. Fat is a choice.

# The
# Secret Lives
# of
# Fat People

# 1

# The Secrets

*"My whole life is centered on food. It's
all I ever think about."*

ALL OF US, fat or thin or in between, have secret parts of
our lives, thoughts and acts that we prefer no one else know
about. In addition to these private guilts, fat people carry
an extra load of secrets. They have more to hide than others
do — secrets that center around eating and weight. These
concern the way they look and feel about themselves, the
amounts and kinds of food they eat, and the lies they tell
themselves and others about being fat.

One of the reasons for keeping such secrets is the delusion
that you do not look as fat as you are. Inside your head is
a vision of a mythical thin person that you would like to
keep alive, a slimmer you that you like to think other people
see. To feed the myth (and your self-esteem), you build
a protective structure around it, a network of other secrets.

These secrets dominate your life.

## What Weight?

Of all the secrets you are most fearful of having discovered,
there is one that you bury deeper than any of the others —

the secret of the exact amount you weigh. That number, whether it is 140, 183, 217, or 312, is your most closely guarded secret. It would be the most terrible event in the world if anyone should find out. It is something even *you* would rather not know. A number is exact, final, and uncompromising. There is no quibbling about it. By revealing it, you destroy the myth.

## Keeping Your Weight a Secret Is Part of Your Fat Problem

I have often asked the people who come to me for therapy how much they weigh. I have never received a straight answer. No one has ever said, "I weigh 184," or even, "I'm over 200 pounds." Instead I have heard, "I don't know. I've stopped weighing myself." Or, "I don't own a scale." Or, "I'm not sure." Sometimes I hear, "I really don't want to talk about it," and, "I don't want to tell you." Some answers are so evasive, it almost seems as if I had asked an entirely different question: "I just lost some weight. I can tell by the way my clothes feel." And, "I've just gone on a diet and I haven't weighed myself yet."

Actually, there are very few people who would risk asking fat people their weight. Even a close friend shies away from such an intimate question. It is potentially too upsetting. It's like asking people how much money they make or asking a no-longer-young movie star how old he or she is. It touches a nerve. And you, the fat person, know this. You depend on it. You enlist the silent aid of others in keeping your secret. After all, if something is a secret, nothing need be done about it. If no one knows how much you weigh, you don't have to lose any weight.

## Invisible Flesh

Not only won't you tell how much you weigh, you won't even admit that you are fat. When new clients come to me, they always begin by explaining the pressing problem that led them to seek therapy. Not once has that pressing problem been fat. Never has a fat person walked into my office and said, "I'm fat. I'm not getting what I want out of life. I was skipped over for a promotion in my job. I can't find a lover. I feel ugly. I want you to help me to lose weight."

After seeing a great many fat people, all of whom behaved as if their flesh were invisible, I began to realize that I was being subtly manipulated away from talking about fat. That I risked incurring the hostility of the fat person. So I waited and wondered when the subject was going to come up. It never did. *I* always brought it up. There is no graceful or gentle way to phrase the query. The question I usually ask is: "How do you feel about being fat?" The response is always the same: surprise — shock, almost — and then silence. Sometimes tears. The nonverbal message is clear: "We can talk about anything. Almost anything. I am open to all subjects but one, and that is the subject of what I weigh or anything related to it. That is my secret. If I want to, *I* will bring it up, not you."

One woman told me, "Asking that question was a direct assault. I felt as if my mother had attacked me physically."

## The Forbidden Subject

To many fat people, merely mentioning the subject of fatness is a form of criticism — criticism that cannot be faced.

Instead, they pretend; they behave as if they were the victim of a congenital defect, like a clubfoot, that has never been corrected. Anyone who brings up fatness is guilty of a gross breach of manners and taste.

While writing this book, I ran into a fat friend whom I had not seen for some time. In the course of catching up with each other's lives, I told her I was writing about fat people. Something odd came over her face when she heard the word *fat*. She sat very still. She didn't blink. She asked no questions, expressed no interest. She didn't say a single word. There was absolutely no response. As I explained what the book was about, I had the eerie feeling that she had shut off all her senses and wasn't there at all — that she was in a state of suspended animation. It was very disconcerting. A great distance opened between us. I quickly changed the subject. Neither of us mentioned the obvious connections: that she was fat, that she had a great deal to say about it, that she could help me with my book, that my book might help her. Hers was a very effective defense against the possibility of my saying something about her weight.

## Even Your Best Friend Won't Tell You

When fat people let it be known implicitly that there are subjects not to be discussed, they draw friends into a conspiracy with them, so that everybody around them is keeping secrets.

At one group therapy session of both thin and fat people, Dick, who weighs over 200 pounds, talked about his friend Mike, who never says a word to Dick about Dick's weight problem. "Mike always tells me that I look great." Al, a thin member of the group, picked up on this. "What kind of a friend is that? A real friend would say something." Al didn't understand that a friend, "real" or not, is often afraid of jeopardizing the friendship with unwanted criticism. Your weight makes him feel too uncomfortable.

## Euphemisms

There is something very harsh about the word FAT, something too realistic to face. It is a word I very rarely hear fat people use. Thin people almost never use it when in the presence of fat people. Another word often avoided is *obese*.

Euphemisms are a form of concealment, a nice way of saying something unacceptable. They blur the truth, present it in a softer light, veil its meaning. What better way to hide your fat than to call it by another name, to cloak it in a gentler phrase? Fat people aren't fat — they're chubby, overweight, a little heavy, plump, portly, heavyset, large-boned, wide-hipped, broad-shouldered, or zaftig.

*Comfortable* is another word fat people like to use a lot. *Comfortable* usually turns out to be a code word for "lazy," for being unwilling to change old habits, especially eating habits. Comfortable eaters are overeaters. Comfortable foods are heavy, filling foods, warm foods, soft foods, baby foods. Comfortable dinners are mashed potatoes with butter and gravy, macaroni and cheese, gooey cake and ice cream.

•

Claire, who is obese, says, "I just shudder when I'm equated with being fat. I don't even like to hear that word. I'm chunky, or solid, or voluptuous... I really know I'm fat, but I don't want to know. Being fat means you're not like other people. If you make the lie big enough, you believe it."

## Rose-colored Glasses

Since fat people won't admit to themselves that they are fat, they also imagine that other people aren't aware of it either. If you don't believe it, it isn't true. You don't really believe that the first thing people notice about you is your fat. You think that people notice your eyes or your smile or your beautiful face. You think the bulky overcoat camouflages your pot belly, the voluminous folds of the tent dress cause fifty pounds or so discreetly to disappear. Once, as I was walking down the street with a fat friend, we passed another equally fat woman. "Do I look like her?" my friend asked me. What she really meant was, "I'm not as fat as that woman, am I?" She would not let herself believe she was "that" fat.

## Ignoring the Obvious

Penny, who is thirty-eight and weighs over 180 pounds, had a date with Neal, who is twenty-six and slim. They had a good time, but he never called again. Penny couldn't understand why. It never occurred to her that her weight was the reason. "We were supposed to go out again, but he canceled at the last minute. He sounded funny — I didn't quite believe his excuse. Later, I found out that he really didn't want to go out with me, but he didn't know how to tell me. I had given him every opportunity. He could have said no, he didn't want to go out. He just couldn't be honest and say that it was because he's younger."

## The Silent Treatment

When the conversation turns to diets, have you ever thought about the guarded way you react? Sometimes you resort to majestic silence (a whiff of hurt feelings ruffling the air), choosing to contribute nothing at all — which makes everyone else nervous and anxious to change the subject. In that way, you manage to manipulate everyone into feeling guilty about bringing up such a sensitive matter — about making *you* feel uncomfortable.

When the conversation shifts to another subject, everyone is off the hook — especially you. Because you aren't able to face your fat, you make sure that no one else does, either.

When you do join the conversation, you usually offer excuses. You can be virtually certain that everyone will be too polite to gainsay you. "I can't stay on a diet," you say, or, "It didn't work for me." Both these phrases imply that the diet is at fault, or that you couldn't stay on it because *it* did something that threw you off. Another popular expression is, "I was doing all right, and then I fell off," as though the surface of the diet were slippery. You come up with all sorts of ingenious reasons for not losing weight. Glands. A sluggish thyroid. Low metabolism. Too many fat cells. Bad genes. Whatever the reason, you are the virtuous one and the victim; the blame lies elsewhere. The excuses mask the real secret — that you aren't really trying; you don't really want to take the trouble to lose weight, and you don't want anyone to know.

## Secret Eating

"I like to eat alone because there is no one to put guilt on me," said Vernon, an obese man. "You eat to the point where you really don't feel good, but it's part of the kick."

Not to be confused with going on a binge, secret eating is the secret of staying fat. It is one of the ways fat people can go on a diet and still succeed in not losing weight. "I just lost ten pounds," your friend tells you excitedly on the telephone, and when you see him he's as fat as ever. Is he lying?

Probably. Lying about food is the connective tissue that holds the whole network of secrets together. I recently shared a hotel room on a business trip with an obese colleague who said she was trying to lose weight. We took our meals together, and at every meal she ate less than I did. She teased me: "Soon you'll weigh more than I do," she said, sipping tea and watching me eat my dessert. One night she left her purse open on the dresser. In it were two candy bars and a cellophane-wrapped Danish pastry. True to the code, I never said a word.

There's the man who eats rabbit food when he's having lunch with co-workers — and keeps a secret cache of candy bars in a drawer of his desk. Nobody can understand why he stays fat. There's the woman who always eats broiled fish and never touches dessert when she's having dinner in a restaurant — and goes home and gorges on chocolate cake. There are all those thousands of people who can't resist the midnight raid on the refrigerator — the chicken salad sandwich dripping mayonnaise, stolen in the middle of the night. And there's the person who doesn't eat regular meals at all, just little snacks between meals — his day becomes one long, endless meal. Rick has the one-meal-a-day delusion: "Yesterday I had pancakes and syrup for breakfast, but all during the day I had pretzels and a couple of ice cream cones and I forget what, and I didn't think of them as a meal. I just had one meal."

## Memory Lapse

When a fat person seems to be only half listening, when her mind seems to be wandering, when she's bored, she's thinking about food. As a fat person, you have food on your mind almost all of the time. As soon as breakfast is over, you begin thinking about what you're going to have for lunch. After lunch, it's time to think about dinner, or stocking the refrigerator for tomorrow. In view of your virtual obsession with food, it's ironic how forgetful you can become. Marcia is on a strict diet and eats only what she is supposed to at meals, but she forgets to remember all the raisins and peanuts she packs away between meals. Ted, also on a diet, seems to go blank during the few minutes when he stops into a McDonald's for a quick fix.

## What Calories?

Everyone with a weight problem is aware of the calorie count of most foods. But you keep secrets from yourself; you play a numbers game with calories. Bob thinks it's fine to eat as much fruit as he wants — apples, grapes, bananas — whatever is in season. The average apple has 90 calories. Bob doesn't let himself be aware of that. If it's fruit it can't be fattening.

Karl won't touch a potato (90 calories) but will put away a thick two-pound steak for dinner. He doesn't think meat is fattening.

•

Margaret adores pasta and eats it twice a day. "Pasta isn't fattening," she says. "Models eat it." Margaret thinks that if it isn't sweet, it doesn't count.

•

Luke won't drink Coca-Cola because of the calories, but he goes through a container of orange juice every day. He refuses to believe orange juice has calories.

•

Suzanne never drinks milk, but she eats two containers of yogurt for lunch.

•

Denise doesn't count *anything* liquid (including Coca-Cola, orange juice, and milk) because "liquids aren't fattening. They're liquid."

•

John has a big lunch and no dinner, but he stops at a bar after work for a couple of drinks — and a few peanuts and pretzels. "When they have potato chips I go crazy, so I avoid that side of the bar. I do drink a lot, but I never count the calories in drinks. I don't believe there are any."

•

Edward puts Sweet 'n Low in his coffee, along with a generous serving of heavy sweet cream. The Sweet 'n Low makes him feel virtuous.

•

Other varieties of calorie blindness are rampant among the fat population:

Toasted bread is less fattening than untoasted bread.

Food eaten at night is more fattening than food eaten during the day.

Cold foods have fewer calories than hot foods.

Bananas are very fattening.

Margarine and cheese are not fattening.

Barbecued spareribs have so little to eat on them that they're not fattening.

If you eat grapefruit twice a day, you'll lose weight.

It's important for health reasons to eat three meals a day.

## Bulimarexia

The latest shameful secret to come to light is the vomiting syndrome known as bulimarexia. Throwing up deliberately is not really a new practice. It was an ancient Roman custom that proved very effective for serious eaters. In the middle of gorging themselves at feasts that went on for days, Romans who were unequal to the occasion would go to a special room called a vomitorium and throw up everything they had just eaten. This enabled them to return to the table with an empty stomach and start eating all over again.

Today's practitioners are more interested in staying thin than in eating a second or third dinner. Just as anorexia nervosa is mainly the province of adolescent girls, so bulimarexia is largely confined to attractive young adult women, many of whom have successful professional careers. No one would perceive them as being fat. They are rarely more than fifteen to twenty pounds overweight. Some are slim but think of themselves as fat or live in terror of becoming fat. They appear to lead normal lives but have a low self-image.

•

Fran, who is 5 feet 5 inches and weighs 118 pounds, is a corporation executive who works under conditions of enormous stress, much of it self-imposed. Although her colleagues think highly of her work, Fran believes that nothing she does is quite good enough. She is a perfectionist. Two or three times a week after work she stops at a grocery store and loads up with candy, cookies, cake, and ice cream, which she devours on her arrival home. Immediately after the binge, before the food has a chance to be digested, she goes to her bathroom and sticks her finger down her throat. "I feel serene afterward, as if all my problems had been solved. I feel in control."

## Clothes

Many fat people look for clothes that will hide the fat, or clothes that will maintain them in the delusion that the fat does not exist. Women drape themselves in nunlike amorphous attire so that no one can see where they leave off and the clothes begin. Such clothing not only blurs the body's outline but lulls the wearer into thinking she is thinner than she really is. It's all an elaborate charade, of course. Thin people wear tight-fitting clothes to show off their bodies, but fat people are convinced that no one can see theirs. Loretta, who comes to me for therapy, wears the same black polyester pants and black smock every time I see her. "When I shop for clothes, I'm so unhappy with what I see in the mirror that I never buy anything," she says. "In these clothes, nobody can tell what I really look like."

One of the most common subterfuges of women who are self-conscious about their fat is to wear clothes that are one or two sizes too big. Caftans, tent dresses, large tops, over-size sweaters are very much a part of an overweight woman's wardrobe. Natalie says, "You think you're inconspicuous wearing tents, when in fact you're this beached whale lumbering through the stores. You think that no one sees your body because you wear makeup and you try to keep a low profile, but meanwhile your *tuches* is knocking over shelves. In one of my classes, a woman walked in, a two-ton. She knocked over the podium, she bumped into the professor, but she was wearing a tent dress and thought that no one saw her."

There are no "fat" fashions to accommodate men, no long flowing robes or loose smocks to hide under, though some wear loose, pleated trousers.

.

Herb is happiest when cold weather comes. "In the winter I can wear nice big bulky Nordic sweaters and vests. In the summer I can't really hide my body. I never wear clingy shirts. The other kind you can sort of blouse up and nobody notices. What's so frustrating is that the styles I like are more for men who wear tight-fitting pants. I have to pick myself up and go to the Arnold Palmer section for middle-aged men. I feel like such a shmuck. I want to be where the disco clothes are, not in the Arnold Palmer Club."

## Shoes

Fat people have all sorts of theories about gravity. One is that shoes with heels lift the body. That is, heels prevent the fat from moving downward and making you look heavier as it seems to do when you wear flat-heeled shoes. High heels give you the illusion that you can hold your posture and carriage together and look thinner.

•

Enid is slender and tiny and looks as though she has never had to worry about her weight. She is one of those people that you think can eat anything and never gain a pound. She says, "When I was heavier, I always wore high heels to make me look taller. That way, the fat would be evenly distributed. When I got thin, buying a pair of flat-heeled shoes was the biggest thing in my life. I had to convince myself that I really didn't look like an egg or a little mushroom in flat shoes. It's hard to change those old feelings."

## Mirrors

When you pass a mirror, it's natural to stop and look at yourself, either to primp or to check yourself out. But mirrors are anathema to fat people. The way you look is something you would rather not come to grips with. When you look deliberately into your own mirror, you don't really see what the mirror is showing you. The view is familiar, and you see the same thing over and over again. You become adjusted to what you are accustomed to seeing. It begins to look "not so bad." When you unexpectedly catch a glimpse of yourself in an unfamiliar mirror, the results are shocking.

•

Ellie says, "I dim the lights before I prepare myself to look in the mirror, and I rarely do it nude. The other day, I walked into the gym where there are mirrors all over the place, and all of a sudden I saw this person. She didn't look familiar. She looked grotesque. It was me. That was the first time that it really hit me, how disgusting I looked."

## Scales

Fat people have a special relationship with scales. Scales are the enemy. Scales are not to be trusted. In a fat person's life, there is no such thing as an accurate scale. They're always a few pounds off, one way or another. One woman I see insists that there is a medical conspiracy: all doctors' scales, she says, are adjusted five pounds upward to make patients believe they are overweight. In your own house, the scales seem to be marked only with numbers that end in five or zero. When you lose weight, you lose five pounds or ten pounds, never two or three or six. The in-between numbers don't count. Three pounds become five by wishful thinking. Fudging the numbers makes them sound better, and the margin for error is reasonable enough not to make it an outright lie.

.

Maryanne creeps up on her scale and tries to surprise it. She gets on very gently, one foot at a time, so the marker moves slowly and doesn't go all the way up before coming back down again. "I figured slow was less. I was sure it was wrong, even when I got on slowly. It always came out the same, but one time I felt really much thinner. I felt I wasn't as fat as people were telling me I was. I got on the scale and bounced — but it didn't go any lower. I started thinking that maybe it was right, and I'd have to face it."

## Fat and Thin

Thin people are endowed by fat people with magical qualities, which render them immune to the daily struggle against putting on weight. The law of life in this fantasy is that the thin person can eat chocolate creams until the end of time and never gain an ounce, while the fat person has only to look at the candy box to gain five pounds. This mysterious ability engenders a great deal of anger and resentment against thin people, resentment that is compounded by the undeniable fact that thin people have an easier time in life and get more out of it than fat people.

It never occurs to fat people that thin people stay thin for a reason. They don't notice that thin people work at staying thin. It doesn't just happen.

•

Irma, who is obese, took a group of friends to lunch at a kosher delicatessen that she often patronizes. Among her friends was a beautiful, slender woman whom Irma particularly resented. Everyone ordered pastrami on rye, french fries (with ketchup), and celery tonic. Irma felt embarrassed about the french fries, but everyone else was having them, so she did too. Irma was so absorbed in her food and her resentment that she failed to observe that the beautiful slender woman ate only the pastrami, not the bread, in order to justify eating a few of the french fries.

## Magical Thinking

Some people come to therapy and say that they have a problem, thinking that it will go away without their working at it. They have an almost superstitious faith that just mentioning the problem will somehow solve it. Similarly, fat people think their weight will simply dissolve at the right time, or that, miraculously, it won't matter. "I finally met a man I liked, and the first thing I did was gain twelve pounds," said Paula, one of my clients, who weighs, I would guess, over 200 pounds. "I don't know how it happened, but I don't think it's important. I really have a feeling this affair is going to work out."

•

Paula isn't just snuggling up to a fantasy. She really believes in her happy ending, even though nothing concrete has happened to encourage that belief. This is known as magical thinking, a kind of self-induced high or euphoria in which you are utterly convinced that everything is going your way. It's the same feeling gamblers get who sense that tonight they can't lose.

•

Helene, who also weighs over 200 pounds, doesn't want to know she has a body. She does not own a full-length mirror on the theory that if she can't see it, it isn't there. Helene also has a magical solution to losing weight. When she gets down to 199 pounds — under the 200 mark — she is sure that the extra pounds will just zoom off. She is afraid to reach the 200 mark.

## Protecting Your Fat

Secrets are your main lines of defense against taking responsibility for your fat. They help you to keep your weight on by not facing it. Thus, you can easily refuse to do anything about it. In the event that any of your defenses are breached, you have developed a secondary line to counter a direct assault. This line consists of certain stock responses designed to stifle all further inquiry. They protect you against other people:

I tried Weight Watchers and every diet you can think of. None of them seems to work for me.

I'm on a diet, but I just can't seem to lose the weight. I think there's something wrong with my glands.

The holidays are coming, and it's impossible to go on a diet during the party season. Once it's over, I can think seriously about dieting.

The last time I was on a diet, I became so weak and irritable that I realized it was very bad for my health.

I'm taking care of my weight. I've given up drinking because liquor has a lot of calories.

I just gave up smoking, and they told us we would put on a few pounds because of that. So I'm not worrying about my weight just now.

My doctor thinks I have a thyroid problem and wants me to get some tests. I haven't gotten around to it yet.

When I'm ready, I'll do something about my weight. I'm just not ready yet.

# 2

# How Fat People
# Are Perceived by Others

*A woman in a supermarket line said to
me, "You know, you have such a pretty
face. How did you get so fat?" I an-
swered, "I worked very hard at it. It
took me a long time to get this way."*

VERY OFTEN, I get a strong sense of the person on the
other end of the telephone who is calling to make an appointment for the first time. I visualize the person physically from voice clues — the tone, the diction, the choice
of words. Occasionally I guess right, as in the case of a
timid frightened voice that later appears as a person to be
the same way.

I have never guessed right when the person on the other
end of the telephone is obese. There is no way of recog-
nizing a fat voice. There is no such thing as a fat voice, nor
is there a fat profile — characteristics psychologists can
pinpoint as belonging to fat people. Yet we all have pre-
conceived notions about fat people. Thin people and fat
people alike are deeply prejudiced against fat people. "He's
nice, but he's so fat," one thin person will say to another,
and they both understand certain biases implicit in the

word *fat*. Nothing else need be said. The prejudice, like those against race, religion, sex, age, or nationality, is often disguised with a friendly, tolerant attitude and rarely, if ever, discussed.

•

Marian, a thin person, told me, "I don't like looking at ugly people, and I don't like to be seen with them. It embarrasses me. When I'm out with someone fat, I imagine that other people are thinking there's something wrong with me for being friends with such an unattractive person. Fat people are gross and disgusting looking. Why should I be tolerant?"

•

Barry said, "Even when I was fat, I practiced the same discrimination that I was a victim of. I treated fat women like sisters. I didn't want to be seen with a fat girl friend. I wanted someone better."

## Show Biz

When fat people look for public images to identify with, scorn and ridicule are reflected back at them. America's opinion of fat people is probably clearest in the portrayal of them in movies and television. Fat is a joke. Fat people are comedians; they play quirky off-beat characters, secondary or ethnic roles. Through the years, Shelley Winters and Maureen Stapleton have exemplified the ethnic lower-class woman. Ernest Borgnine has performed that function for men.

Even now, when glamour isn't what it used to be, it is hard to find a single young new star who isn't thin. Sex symbols are not fat. When they have a tendency to gain weight, they take care of it fast. Elizabeth Taylor has struggled with a weight problem for years, always having to diet before each new movie. Between acting engagements, she gives up the struggle.

For men, the exceptions to the rule have been geniuses — Marlon Brando, Orson Welles — or those who have enduring box office appeal despite both age and fat — Cary Grant and the late John Wayne, Clark Gable and Gary Cooper. The glamorous female stars of the forties and fifties did not fare so well. Only a handful continue to get good parts — Katharine Hepburn, Lauren Bacall, Audrey Hepburn. All three look bony and fragile.

On television, the overweight male leads of series project a dippy quality. They play character roles, not handsome-leading-men roles. Peter Falk, who plays the dumpy Columbo, rattles on incessantly about his domestic affairs, drives a tacky old car, and has a droopy dog. His raincoat is a wreck, and he is a pest. William Conrad, the fattest of the lot, plays Frank Cannon, a private detective whose bulk had to be justified by turning him into a gourmet cook. His attitude toward women is fatherly. Carroll O'Connor and Jean Stapleton (Archie and Edith Bunker), the essence of ethnicity, are both fat. Not one of these characters exhibits a sign of grace or elegance.

Opera stars have been the sole exception to the ban on fat. Traditionally, they have been overweight. According to the common wisdom, voice resonance depended on weight. As proof, it was said that the late Maria Callas lost her voice when she lost weight. Recently, however, this attitude has changed, at least with regard to female singers. It has come to matter what the prima donna looks like, as well as how she sounds.

## Some Common Views of Fat People

Fat people have no will power. They get fat and stay fat because they are lazy. Inactive, they cause surprise when they ride a bicycle or engage in a sport. There is something physically wrong with them, and therefore they are to be avoided, like freaks. Fat people are sloppy, slovenly, sweaty, smelly. They are incompetent, undisciplined, irresponsible, ignorant. They take up too much space; no one wants to stand or sit next to them. They are uncontrolled. They are sexless, epicene. Fat men are passive and not capable of behaving in masculine ways. Fat women nurture themselves instead of others. Fat people are antisocial. They are to be pitied. They are less than human: they are "other." Socially and sexually, they are no threat to thin people. Fat people are good dancers, light on their feet. They have a good sense of humor and are easy to get along with. They are calm and gentle, good listeners; they are neither mean nor petty. They are flexible in outlook. Fat women have pretty faces.

The kinds of images most of us identify with are of people who are lithe, lean, quick, energetic, slim, young. This is the model advertisements hold up for us — we must be young and vigorous. The images are invested with a moral quality; it is considered "good" to be like that. Fat people, who are clumsy, heavy, slow, and lethargic, are thus obscurely "bad."

These prejudices are indiscriminately attributed to fat people. If a fat man is clumsy, it is assumed that *all* fat men are clumsy. Fat people are not viewed as individuals. They are masses of flesh, indistinguishable from each other.

These prejudices remain unspoken. Other attitudes operate on a more open level and may be even more painful to fat people.

## The Jolly Fat Person

Perhaps the most common myth about fat people is that they are always good-humored, always easygoing and ready to laugh. Because of low self-esteem and feelings of worthlessness, fat people comply with the stereotype; you do what is expected. If you weren't jolly and happy, why would anyone want to bother with you?

·

Audrey, who is always pleasant and patient, says, "I was the one that everyone came to, the confidence taker. People came to me when they wanted to be cheered up. I was good for a laugh, and I helped them sort out their lives. I got tired and bored with other people's problems, but I figured if I didn't listen, they wouldn't want to have anything to do with me."

·

Being jolly is a fat person's ticket to acceptance. It is important that the rest of us think you are happy. If you're happy, there's nothing seriously wrong with you. You're not a freak. The jollity masks your rage and pain, neither of which is acceptable. Humorousness becomes a form of shuffling, something all powerless groups in society feel compelled to accept in order to avoid bringing down the wrath of the powerful on their heads. It's an emotional disguise, even as loose clothes camouflage the physical reality.

·

Les, who was fat until he was thirty years old, says, "I've got a brick wall around me. I'm afraid to get hurt. Very few people get by that brick wall. I just dance and sing and play around, and nobody gets close to me. It's protection. You have to develop protection."

•

Kitty is deeply resentful of the role her fat has cast her in. "I may seem like a fat happy person, but all of my problems go into my mouth. It makes me angry to become a stereotype. I want to say I have problems too. You just never found out about them because I never let them out. I wasn't supposed to. I'm supposed to be a happy, smiling little girl. Always smiling. Someone told me recently, 'I never knew you had problems because you always seem so happy, with a nice smile on your face.' I wanted to kick him."

•

Harvey, a fat child, cultivated jolliness to compensate for not being able to do other things. "I kept trying to be like the other boys. I was never athletic, but I would play ball anyway. I went skating at 300 pounds. I'd fall and get up and hope that people would at least notice that a fat guy could move. I'd make a big production over missing the Frisbee, and then start joking about myself. It took away the pain. When someone else joked about me, it hurt."

## Friendless

When a thin and a fat person seem to be good friends, the thin person is often using the fat person as a backdrop against which he can look better. The fat person, who thinks he is ugly and therefore worthless and inferior, is grateful for the attention. He will go out of his way to do favors for the thin person, as proof of his worthiness and to give the thin person reason to continue to be his friend.

•

Marty, who grew up fat, is bitter when he remembers his childhood and the pain he felt. "People discriminate against you. A group of guys go off to play ball, and you have to invite yourself. You're not automatically included. They know you're not fast. I was always left out, except for the comic relief. When I did play, I always tried to get on the losing team so nobody would be mad at me."

•

Kathleen spends her spare time doing favors for friends who take her for granted and never dream of repaying her. Kathleen thinks so little of herself that she demands nothing in return — and gets nothing. She's a good sport; she's nice; she's helpful. The nicer she is, the more she hates herself. "I work for a film company. A friend of mine asked if she could borrow a film to show to some friends at a party to which I was not invited. I not only was delighted to get it for her, I even told her I'd bring it over to her house to make it easier for her. Why would she want anyone as fat as I am for a friend?"

•

Norman, who is no longer fat, says, "A friend of mine got a little twitchy when my weight dropped below what he weighs. There's social pressure to stay fat. People know how to deal with you; you're the scapegoat."

## Sexless

For the longest time, Paul didn't have to worry about whether people were attracted to him or about sexuality.

"I was like Father Earth, giving out advice and nurturing people. I thought, well, people like me because of that, and why should I worry about sex? I was giving something to people, and that was good enough for me. As soon as I started talking about being gay — as soon as I put sexuality into the conversation — people backed off. Not only couldn't they deal with their homophobia, but suddenly I wasn't Father Earth anymore. I was a sexual person."

## Exploited

"Mary Jane is really brilliant, and she has a beautiful face, but she's a slob, a real slob. She's over 200 pounds. Her boy friend never really sees *her*. He doesn't care what's going on inside her head. He doesn't see her as a person. She's a thing to be used, to cook great meals for him."

•

"Doris thinks that she's a normal weight. Anyway, she acts that way. She's at least 300 pounds. She's always making overtures to men, even with all those things that would really make me vomit — the bad teeth, the odor, and all the weight. It's unreal, that weight. She does get boy friends, but they're the kind who don't want to take her out — you know, just keep-them-in-the-house kind of boy friends. Doris never says that she's gone here or she's gone there; it's, 'Oh well, Vince and I just sit home,' and this woman is only about twenty-seven years old."

## Workless

Like women, minorities, the elderly, and the handicapped, fat people are discriminated against on the job. Few if any employers would care to go on record as saying so, but when there are several candidates for a job, the fat one is least likely to be hired.

.

Helen, young and obese, had the office skills — no one could fault her typing and shorthand. Secretarial jobs were available. After a year of job hunting, she was finally told by the employment agency that employers simply didn't want to look at her. "It shattered me," Helen said. "It's not my fault. I have a thyroid problem." Even if Helen had brought a letter from her doctor, employers still would not have wanted to look at her.

.

Bill, a salesman, was aced out for a promotion because of his fat. His small-town clients enjoyed seeing him — he was jolly and funny and good company. Bill was smart enough to realize he was expected to behave that way, according to his clients' prejudices. His success hinged on it; it helped him consistently to sell more than his quota. If merit had been the only criterion, Bill would have been an executive. "We need you in the field," Bill was told officially. Privately, his boss said, "The New York office is a showcase. He just wouldn't look right there."

.

Many fat people are hidden away in a back room somewhere and passed over for promotions and raises. Among people earning $25,000 a year and up, only 9 percent are overweight. "A fat person would give the company a bad image." "We want someone young and attractive." "Fat people don't appeal to clients." The inability of fat people to get ahead reinforces prejudices against them — they are incompetent, slow-moving, have emotional problems.

Such people, it is thought, cannot be trusted with responsibility. Anyone unable to discipline herself enough to lose weight certainly must be incapable of doing important work. "If they can't control their weight problem, fat people are not totally dependable about other matters."

## Untrusted

If you're fat you're undisciplined; if you're undisciplined you can't be trusted to do anything right. Guilt by association works on the personal level, too. A schoolteacher with a problem child in her class suspected the boy's disruptive behavior stemmed from problems at home. When his mother walked in for a conference, the teacher all but gave up. The mother was grossly overweight, and the teacher immediately assumed a woman like that had too many problems of her own to handle the child's difficulties.

Fat people, who are usually down on themselves to begin with, are certainly not insensitive to the low opinion society holds of them. Sometimes they go so far as to blame everything that goes wrong on being fat. "The waiter was nasty, and I'm sure it was because I'm fat." "When I was heavy, people would shortchange me. I always translated it to mean that they hated fat people. I could never say, 'I gave you a ten, not a five.' I never felt aggressive enough."

To most fat people, the prejudice against them is another secret in the long list of subjects never to be mentioned. Generally, they prefer to ignore it; it's too painful, too humiliating and dehumanizing to confront. However, like other groups that find themselves victimized, some fat people have organized to fight their unpleasant image and the prejudices against them.

## Fat Power

*Big Beautiful Woman*, a new national magazine catering to the overweight, was founded in 1979 by Carole Shaw, a woman who dieted for years and achieved a size 9 "for two days." She said, "I have been on diets since I was eleven, and I have had it. No more dieting for me. It's such a waste of energy."

In the past decade, a new movement of obese people has arisen. Called The National Association to Aid Fat Americans, it is dedicated to the proposition that it's all right to be fat. Members object to the way fat people are perceived, not to being fat. Fat people are fine, the membership insists; it is society that has a problem, and it is the way society treats them that makes fat people unhappy. "I'm unhappy because I'm ostracized from society," a fat woman said. "But in my personal life, I have friends. There are people who love me. I have a social life. I have a good time."

Members of the group appeared on the CBS-News television show, *60 Minutes*, filmed at their 1979 convention in Washington — a weekend of fat pride. Mike Wallace, known for his caustic interviewing technique, was surprisingly gentle with this group — even as the rest of us are intimidated by fat people from speaking out.

WOMAN: I want to be respected, I want to be acknowledged, and I want to be loved for who I am. I don't want to walk down the street and have people turn around and make fun of my package.

WOMAN: Men would like to be with fat women in the open, go to restaurants and everything else, but society has put so much pressure on them, telling them, "Hey, you have to go out to a restaurant with a skinny woman."

WOMAN: A lot of the guys are in the closet about liking fat women. They come here. They're single guys. They don't want their friends to know they're with fat women.

MAN: Some people like me enjoy looking at fat people. I love to look at a fat woman on the beach. If I saw Marilyn Monroe or Gina Lollobrigida on the beach, they'd turn me off. They're like looking at a board.

WOMAN: Clothes are made with no conception of what looks good on a fat woman. Stores use attractive, thin women to model their clothes.

WOMAN: I was in Macy's one day watching girls with big hats hand out perfume samples. You stand there long enough, you never see them hand one to a fat person . . . fat people evidently don't use perfume.

WOMAN: You never see anybody heavy using any product on TV.

WOMAN: Except oven cleaner.

The prejudices with which fat people are perceived and treated have a profound effect on your own behavior and self-image. Because you are so vulnerable to criticism, you inevitably internalize at least some of the prejudices against you. You are thus forced further into holding a damaging view of yourself and your fat, and made more vulnerable and secretive. The secrets soften reality and help you to feel better about your plight.

# 3

# How Fat People
# Perceive Themselves

*"I spend a lot of time wondering how I look and if other people are wondering about how much I weigh."*

FAT PEOPLE are not very easy on themselves. Time and again, I have heard a fat person tell me he thought he looked ugly, disgusting, revolting. Indeed, fat people are probably more judgmental and prejudiced against other fat people than thin people are. They are also the quickest to hate and torment themselves about their own fat. Their attitude is ambivalent. On the one hand, they sympathize with and understand the fat condition; on the other, they see in themselves the traits society attributes to them — the disorder, the self-indulgence, the lack of self-control — and condemn themselves. "Even though I don't change my weight, I do manage to control my emotions," a fat woman said. "I don't like to see such an obvious lack of control in other fat people. I guess it's something I'm saying about myself."

## "I Am Ashamed"

Ordinary things that everyone else does as a matter of course are fraught with shame for fat people and performed in secrecy. "When I was in college, I was ashamed to undress in front of my roommate," Rita said. "I changed under my nightgown. When it was cold, I tried to stay under the covers. Sometimes I changed in one of the stalls in the bathroom. I couldn't bear to let anyone see how I looked."

Maureen has the same feeling with salesclerks. "When I buy clothes, I'm terrified that someone is going to walk into the dressing room and see how fat I am. I never shop with friends. I even feel funny about buying food. I keep thinking that everyone is watching to see what I load into my cart, just waiting to point a finger at me the minute I buy something fattening. I don't even enjoy going out to dinner with my friends. Eating in public is a terrible ordeal. I feel as if everyone is watching every mouthful I take. I'm never sure if I should order what I like or what people think I should be ordering. And dessert! I wouldn't dream of ordering dessert in public."

## Togetherness

Fat people who would not normally be friends are often drawn to each other to compensate for possible rejection from the rest of the world. They form a nonthreatening alliance in which neither person is embarrassed by the other, a mutual support system to indulge in eating orgies together.

You know and you don't want to know how the two of you must look together — and what the basis of the friendship is. "We would kvetch about being overweight and not liking the clothes we were wearing, but at dinner we would order outrageous desserts after a full meal — and we ate every course that came with the dinner," Shelly said.

•

There is something comforting about feeling that the person you are with is in as bad shape as you are or — even better for your own self-image — worse than you. You certainly don't want to compare yourself to someone who always looks good, especially when you feel that you look terrible. Misery loves company. "All my friends were dumpy and fat. When I started making friends with more attractive people, I felt lousy about myself," Ethel said.

•

Daisy says, "All my life I've had fat friends. Maybe they really weren't friends, but that was the way I built relationships. The first time I met Arlene, we started to talk about being overweight and dieting. I had a partner in my eating business. Before Arlene, I had another fat girl friend in the neighborhood. I used to see her all the time, but after I moved and lost weight I never called her, and I realized I couldn't stand her. I'd overlooked her unpleasant personality because of our being able to eat together."

## Competition

It's natural to want to excel at something, to be as good as or better than the next person, and to want to do something well. Fat people are rarely given the opportunity to achieve that kind of competent image of themselves. To make up for it, they sometimes have a compensatory reaction. The one thing a fat person can indisputably be is fatter than someone else. After all, if you're going to be fat, why not be the fattest? On a noontime New York television talk show that featured a discussion of obesity, many fat women in the audience vied with each other to see who weighed more. They seemed to take a perverse pleasure in weighing more than anyone else, like taking the booby prize in a contest. When a woman said she had gone from a size 18 to a size 10, they scoffed at her. You only lost about sixty pounds," they said. "That's not fat."

## The End of a Beautiful Friendship

Two fat friends who had known each other for years decided to go on a diet together. They would each lose twenty pounds a month. Doing it together would make it easier, they reasoned, and the competition would be an incentive to succeed. After three weeks and ten pounds, Bernice threw in the towel. Darlene persevered and lost the twenty pounds — and then went on to lose another twenty. The friendship has never been the same. They rarely see each other anymore, and when they do, Bernice, who weighs more than she did when the bargain was struck, is consumed with envy and resentment. She goes home and eats to make herself feel better.

## Opposites Attract

Although fat people seem to have a great deal in common, they are not often sexually attracted to one another. On the contrary. Like all women, a fat woman wants to be accepted for who she is, not the way she looks; but she doesn't feel the same way about the men she goes out with. She usually likes well-built and good-looking men.

.

Veronica, who weighs close to 170 pounds, recognizes her double standard and is disturbed by it. She doesn't want to be seen with anyone who doesn't make her look good — but going out with an attractive man makes her feel ugly. She prefers to feel ugly. "I used to go out with guys who were definitely pear-shaped, and I thought they looked O.K. in public. Then, when I was watching them undress, I'd say, 'Ugh.' I'm really hung up on bodies. I always thought that if I were in love with a person I could just accept him totally. Forget it. If he's not a certain shape, I won't bother with him. I feel guilty about not being more tolerant."

## Sameness Repels

Alma had a long-term live-in relationship with a man who was as overweight as she. She became disgusted with him and moved out. "I kept gaining and gaining. It took me a long time to realize that we were each feeding ourselves, and nothing was going on between us. My body didn't reject the food because my head was saying, 'Well, I have a real need for it because he's not giving me anything.' He *couldn't* give me anything — he was too busy feeding himself."

.

Often, the very thing that brings fat men and women together is what drives them apart. Jeffrey said, "Mary has a big weight problem. When I was with her for a month or so, I began to see patterns. All of a sudden I thought,

'That's me.' I saw what I did, and it was helpful to me just to observe Mary. I was disgusted with her. If I hadn't seen myself, it wouldn't have bothered me that much."

## Male and Female

Many fat men think women won't mind if they have a beer belly and walk around with fat slopping over the top of their pants. To them, it's a sign of masculinity, of being one of the boys. Gerry said, "I care more about what men think of the way I look. Women go out with me, but when I play tennis with the guys, my stomach embarrasses me."

A man can be twenty or thirty pounds overweight and still be considered eligible. Fat men have less trouble finding dates than fat women. Men have an advantage. Because they are generally taller and broader than women, the extra weight — which is usually concentrated around the middle — doesn't show as much. The fat doesn't look quite so fat on them. "Fat men don't question themselves about coming on to you," a thin woman observed. "It doesn't seem to dawn on them that they're not desirable."

Socially, it is far more important for women to be thin. Men perceive themselves less in terms of looks and more in terms of achievement than women do. Many overweight men allow themselves to become fat when they reach middle age and have already achieved a position in life. The achievement of that position, the confidence and the money and power that go with it, are far more important for sexual success with women than having a thick midsection. Fat or thin, money and power are sexy. "If I put on a lot of weight, I would just have a gut, and if people didn't like it, well, too bad," Patrick said.

Which is not to say that men don't care at all. Men rarely talk about these matters, but a fat man who has been fat since childhood feels the stigma in a way that one who has been accustomed to a life of being thin does not. The man who was once thin has an image of himself as normal and acceptable, and behaves that way; the man who was a fat child still sees himself as fat and unattractive. He has the same preoccupation with body image, the same kinds of worries about flabby flesh as women do. This may come as a surprise to many women who think that self-hatred in fat people is primarily a female problem.

•

Adam, who grew up fat and is now thin and successful at thirty-six, says, "It's hard being fat. Women don't want to go out with you, especially in high school. They don't want to be seen with you because you don't look good. You can't get clothes that fit. You're an outcast when you're growing up. It's like being a leper. I was never invited to the big parties. Later on, you have money, you have a car, you have some decent clothes, but it's still hard to get over the bad times you've had. You become very self-reliant. I don't need anybody anymore. I can be happy by myself. You have to entertain yourself. You have to use your imagination. I love movies, I love TV, I like fantasy. It's a good way to stay away from painful situations."

## Clothes

Fat people dress to accomplish one of two opposing purposes — to camouflage or to be conspicuous.

•

"There are certain clothes that fat people shouldn't wear," said Brenda. "Like tight sweaters. I have a load of size 40 sweaters, shapeless, to cover me up. I have navy A-line dresses with white collars and cuffs. No matter how fat I am, you can't tell."

•

Grace sticks with dark colors — black and brown in winter, and navy blue in summer. "I spend more energy camouflaging than I do losing weight."

•

Ernie always wears a loose shirt at the beach. "People tell me to take off my shirt, and I tell them I burn easily. I'd love to take my shirt off, but I can hardly bear to look at myself without clothes, so how can I expect anyone else to?"

•

Jane, who has two children, has been divorced for eight months and has let herself get forty-two pounds heavier than she was the last time she saw her ex-husband, who looks trim and fit. When he comes to pick up the children, she usually sends them downstairs alone. Once, he wanted to speak with her. She panicked. "I really didn't want him to see me so fat. I had this Sherlock Holmes hat that I pulled over my head. I wore a long pea green trench coat, and I put on slacks. I looked terrible, but I didn't look as if I had gained forty-two pounds."

•

Fat people who wear bright colors and splashy prints take a more metaphysical approach to hiding their bodies. They reason that they want to emphasize their face and eyes. Brilliant colors do indeed reflect brighter faces.

•

Holly, a young college student, always wears bright-colored turtleneck sweaters, which expand the width and depth of her body and emphasize her large breasts. One day she came in wearing a loose black top with a V-neck. She looked twenty pounds lighter. When I told her how becoming it was, she said, "I couldn't find anything in my closet that fits since I've been binging so much, so I put this on even though I think black looks terrible on me. I don't understand it — my boss asked me if I'd lost weight. In fact, I've gained."

## Not Caring

"When I feel fat I feel ugly, and it doesn't matter what I look like," said Yvonne. "I wear just any old thing. There was a time when I wouldn't wear pants because I thought they made me look too fat. Now I wear them all the time. I look grotesque — but whatever I wear I look grotesque."

•

Andy hates to get dressed. "On weekends, I loll around the house in my pajamas until three o'clock in the afternoon. Then I go out — to buy food."

•

Pamela, whose weight goes up and down, says, "When I'm losing weight, I take care of everything. You can tell just by walking into my apartment that I'm dieting. I'm not talking about what's in the refrigerator. My apartment is clean. My clothes are ironed. My hair is washed. When I'm a big fat slob, I don't even set my hair or do my face. I don't want to call attention to myself."

## Top Heavy

Many fat women feel particularly self-conscious about their large breasts.

•

Ingrid was thin but overdeveloped as a teenager. "When I was fourteen, I was fourteen going on twenty-one. I just had to flatten myself out. My mother bought me big brassieres, the ones that go from your stomach practically to your armpits, and I used to walk around hugging myself. Today I'm a 34-B and I'm still self-conscious about being too big. I'm not, but I think I am. I read an ad for a new kind of bra that makes you look smaller, and I'm going to buy it."

•

Being big-breasted is not only a matter of weight but of proportion.

•

"I always thought I would never have a good body because I'm out of proportion," Roslyn said. "It was only recently that I could be a decent weight, but I still don't feel O.K. about my body. By my standard of beauty, no matter how much weight I lose I still feel really busty."

## Shyness

Often a fat person is hesitant about meeting new people.

•

"I'm shy," Bruce says, but he isn't shy; he just doesn't want to be the only fat person in the group.

•

After years of having a terrible time at parties, Ina has sworn off them. "When I enter a room full of people I've never seen before or who don't know me, I want to merge into a wall. I start wishing I were invisible. If they know me it's O.K. because they know I'm funny and nice. If they don't know me, I feel that they're judging me strictly on my looks which, to put it mildly, are not wonderful. That's when I really know I'm fat."

## Anger

All fat people don't just pull in their horns and meekly accept their inferior position. Sometimes pussycats are transformed into angry lions. Refusing to be rejected, they deliberately use their anger as a weapon, knowing their size and bulk can easily intimidate people. To some big strong overweight people, pounds equal power.

.

A St. Louis, Missouri, gas station attendant said, "Well, nobody treats me bad because I weigh 275 pounds, and I don't take no lip from nobody."

.

Violet, who is 5 feet 8 inches and weighs over 300 pounds, says, "As a fat kid I was always bigger than anyone else. People used to tease me, and I developed a fast mouth. That's what happens. You go one of two ways. Either you slink back into yourself and become accommodating, or you develop a fast mouth. The kids in the neighborhood were really mean to me. So I started telling them about their physical disabilities — all the things I thought were wrong with them. They stopped being mean."

## Confusion

Many fat people lack a sure sense of how they look, believing either that they are fatter or thinner than they really are.

·

"I had a salad for lunch, and I just know I looked thin after I ate it," an obese man said. Having used self-control, he thought it showed.

Sometimes the image is left from another time in your life.

·

Lindsay, a fat child who is now thin, wears big, loose shirts. Twenty years after the fact, she still thinks of herself as fat and keeps trying to hide the weight that isn't there anymore.

·

Karen, thirty years old, who has been both fat and thin, says, "When I was a child, shopping was a big expedition. First we'd get my sister's clothes, and then we'd go to the chubbette department. I had to get little tent dresses. I always looked like a fat frump. After I lost weight in college, I would go straight to the size 14s. I just assumed that 14 was my size, that I was still a nine-year-old chubbette."

·

Melvin, who is no longer fat, still lives with his old fat self. "I was in economics class and the professor remarked that people should be taxed by their weight. Instinctively, I said, "I resent that." He looked at me in a puzzled way and asked why. I realized I had lost seventy pounds. I was still reacting as if I were fat."

## Looking Backward

Vanessa's vision of herself is colored by regret and stalled in the past. She wants desperately to have been something other than what she was, to live a part of her life again. "I was very heavy in high school; that was my heaviest time. I used to fantasize about going to my reunion, ten years later. When it came, I weighed about twenty-five pounds less, and I was a couple of inches taller. I didn't have my braces anymore and wore contact lenses. I decided to go back. I went back in a prom dress, thinking I looked ten years younger than anybody else there. I didn't go back as a woman; I went back in the image that I wanted to have when I was in high school."

·

As a fat person, you are an outsider in a thin society. If you lived alone on a desert island, if fatness were suddenly to become fashionable, if thinness were viewed as abnormal or unsexy, you would be more attractive in other people's eyes and your own. You would still feel physically uncomfortable, sweat heavily, be out of breath, not fit in chairs, be clumsy at sports — but so would everyone else.

The images in your head of how you look and your attitudes about fat are derived from the way other people view you. The shame, the self-hatred, the ambivalence toward other fat people are your direct responses to your situation. But they are also *your* attitudes; they come from *your* head.

How did you get into this situation, and how can you get out of it?

# 4

# Raising Fat Children
# to Be Fat People

*"I put a lot of blame for being fat on my family. They didn't teach me good eating habits."*

"THERE WERE ALWAYS FIGHTS at the dinner table. My sister got lots of attention and was yelled at and punished because she was a fussy eater. I ate everything and even asked for more so that I would be the good one."

•

"The atmosphere around the table was always tense because my dad would read the paper while he ate. He wouldn't talk to us. My mother would criticize his table manners, and we would try to get some attention from him, but we were continually ignored. I would gobble my food quickly, and just as quickly leave the table."

•

"My parents worked. They left money for me on the kitchen table so that I could buy anything I wanted to eat. That was the beginning of my loneliness eating. I got out of school at noon and bought candy, cakes, anything I wanted. When my mother came home, she would ask me if I had bought a sandwich and fruit or anything like good food. I'd always lie and say I had."

·

"Dinner time was just awful. My parents were very strict about table manners. If I did something sloppy like put my elbows on the table or forget to change my fork from my left hand to my right, I would be instantly corrected. Sometimes I was ordered to leave the table in the middle of dinner and go to my room until I learned better manners. So I began my sneaky eating — raiding the refrigerator when no one could see me."

·

"Even though my family was well off, my mother just didn't believe in buying too much food. There was one hamburger apiece and no seconds. The soda was evenly divided, never quite enough to fill up a glass. We would all watch each other greedily and jealously. Now I like to have plenty of food available so that I can eat as much as I want."

·

"I loved eating at friends' houses when I was a kid. They always had wonderful things to eat that we never had. I still love eating at other people's houses. Maybe the food wasn't really that wonderful, but to me anything was better than eating at home. The atmosphere was more relaxed. At home, eating was always a big deal. My mother didn't believe in pampering us. My friends always had real chocolate milk that came in a bottle instead of the kind where you have to put in the syrup yourself and mix it. My mother said it was too expensive and that I was such a greedy pig, I couldn't be trusted not to drink the whole thing myself, since I didn't like sharing with my brother and sister."

·

"I used to be ashamed of my father at the table. Gross, that's the only word I can think of. He ate with such passion. And he was very sloppy. He and my mother never got along, and she was disgusted by him at the dinner table. They had their biggest fights right after dessert. The arguments wouldn't be about food, though. They'd be about anything. I always felt sorry for Dad, even though it was such a turnoff to watch him eat. I think it was his only pleasure. Today I'm probably just as fat as he was, but I do all my heavy eating in private. I'm probably just as much of an animal when I stuff myself, but I won't let anyone see me."

.

The fat adult is simply a fat child who became older. If you sometimes think of yourself as a child — particularly when you feel an uncontrollable desire to eat something — do you also feel, even momentarily, that you have abdicated responsibility for your life?

While other aspects of your personality have matured, some of your eating habits have not. In the patterns that were set up during infancy and childhood, you were the powerless one. That feeling may still be there. Although you may be in control of other areas of your life, the old emotional tensions of eating may never have been completely resolved.

Those early dinner scenes, enlightening as they are, are not the root of your food problem. They illustrate certain eating patterns that grew out of even earlier experiences. Food problems begin long before any conscious memory of them. They begin in infancy.

I don't believe that discovering the "why" or "how" of your fat problem will make the problem go away. There are no miracles. There is no such thing as a quick flash of insight when suddenly everything changes and the extra pounds slide away forever. Losing weight doesn't work like that. But I do believe it is helpful to relive some of those early traumas about food and meals. They are a clue to the mystery of how old patterns continue; they are a way of assessing the damage and seeing what you can do about it.

## The Helpless Infant

Almost all your overeating is irrational eating. You don't know why you do it. You have a vague sense of emptiness inside; you feel somehow deprived. You don't exactly know what it is you feel deprived of — the feeling is too vague to pin down — but there seems to be some solace in filling that empty space inside. You know at least that it isn't food you feel deprived of — but what is it?

The feeling is the same one you once had when you were a hungry infant lying in the crib, waiting for someone to feed you or comfort you. It is a feeling of helplessness.

Infants have only one way of signaling their needs — by crying. The very young infant feels herself to be part of the person (an indistinct object) who takes care of her. To gain power over this person, the infant cries and she is fed or touched. As Dr. Nathan Ackerman observed in his book, *The Psychodynamics of Family Life*, in the infant's view "the child commands, the mother obeys ... the mother functions as a source of love and security ..." The way in which parents respond to an infant's cries is crucial. The infant cannot separate her needs and cannot explain whether she is hungry or wants to be held. She knows only that she needs, and she cries. The parents' response helps her focus on exactly what it is she wants and helps her learn to feel content when her needs are filled.

Some parents are highly sensitive to their baby's cries, able to distinguish among the need to be fed, changed, turned over, held, and comforted. Such parents usually do not stick to a rigid feeding schedule but rely on the baby's inner clock. "Watch the baby, not the clock," one family physician has cautioned.


## Instant Gratification

When the infant's needs are taken care of without his having to wait too long, he becomes confident of himself and his world. The older the baby gets, the longer he is able to wait for the fulfillment or gratification of his needs. He has had the experience of satisfaction during that very early period. The parents have helped him to know what he wants and have given him the sense that his needs will continue to be fulfilled when they arise. He has emotional and biological confidence.

Fat adults also want to experience instant gratification.

·

Ruth said, "I can't seem to put off gratification at all. Whether it's food or a hug or sex, when I want it, I want it. I sit obsessed throughout the day about what I don't get and why I am not getting it and who is not giving it to me, and I'm depressed. That's why I'm in therapy. I can't picture what life would be like without plotting and manipulating to get somebody to fill the vacuum."

## Overfeeding

Some parents may overfeed a baby, thinking (after checking to see that a diaper pin hasn't opened) that every cry is a hunger cry. There may even be a competition in the family among those who feed the baby. "See how much she eats for me." Food is often offered as the universal panacea, the cure for all discomfort. In such families, it is unthinkable that a child be unhappy, for that would reflect on the parents. "A fat baby is a happy baby," is such a family's maxim.

## Confusion

When food is the great pacifier, offered to cure the discomforts of everything from a stomachache to a wet diaper, a child comes to distrust the validity of her own feelings and body signals. The result is a person who cannot distinguish between feeling hungry and feeling unhappy. In extreme cases, some obese adults are haunted by the fear of starvation. The child is merely confused. Love and approval are mixed up in her head. She equates eating with happiness and love and not eating with disapproval. "All gone," are two of the earliest words in our vocabulary, spoken with joy and triumph. The child, and later the adult, develops a destructive relation with food, using it to solve problems that are not related to eating. The fat adult is a fat child who is still confused about her own body signals and feelings. The fat adult stuffs herself as a quick and easy way to gain love.

## Frustration

In every family, there are times when no one knows why the baby is crying or how to comfort him, and other times when no one comes to pick him up. Someone says, "Let the baby cry; it's good exercise for his lungs." The baby is screaming away, red in the face, enraged at receiving no response. (Remember, he feels omnipotent; his natural expectation is that someone will come and take care of him.) He waits and waits and finally begins to feel that no one will ever come, that his source of love and security — and food — has dried up. The child, even as early as a month or two of age, has feelings of helplessness, rage, panic, and apathy.

When an infant screams for a long time, the parents become angry and frustrated. *They* begin to feel helpless, and they resent it. They are determined that the child will not control their lives. "We will not jump every time he screams." So the conflict begins, initiated by the parents' response to the infant. Frustration builds. This is the beginning of a person's insecurity about being fed or comforted. A pattern for eating is established that continues in childhood at the dinner table. Fearful of not getting enough (or any), a child tries to get as much as he can. As adults, different events may trigger the same emotional response in us. We continue in the same old pattern — trying to fill the emptiness — unaware of the trigger.

## Rewards and Punishments

Later, as a child gets older, food is used for control, for some purpose other than eating. Food carries an emotional load quite beyond its content. The parents exercise control by a system of rewards and punishments. The most common situation is having to eat food you dislike in order to be rewarded with dessert. You really don't like those vegetables, or maybe you're just too full to finish them. You complain, you fight, but you get them down anyway, for the sake of the cake. As an adult, you continue to reward yourself in the same manner, forgetting how it all began.

Sooner or later, the incredible revelation comes: you can now have as many desserts as you want. You become an overpermissive parent to yourself. "*Now* no one can tell me how much or how little I can have. *Now* I can eat all I want. I am finally the boss."

## Problem Eaters

The child exercises control by choosing to eat, not eat, or overeat. She forces her parents to pay attention, and she makes them jump. Most of the time what she is doing is unconscious, not a carefully thought out wicked plot. She is making sure she doesn't need anyone to feed her, that dependence having already proved unreliable. She puts herself in charge of eating, overfeeding herself in order not to feel deprived. She knows she will get a reaction if half the cake is missing from the refrigerator.

Any attention — even yelling — is better than none. As an adult, your eating behavior parallels that of your childhood. Most of the time the parallels remain hidden, a secret even from you.

Trish, a thirty-seven-year-old client, told me, "Usually I buy Life Savers and a Hershey bar before I come to see you. I eat the Hershey bar as I walk up the stairs. I know you know, and I really want you to yell at me. If you yelled and said, 'You know you don't need it,' I would feel good. My mother did that to me all the time. But you don't say anything. You just look at me. I'm sure you care, but if you *really* cared, you'd yell at me. I feel childish trying to hide candy from you, and I want you to disapprove of me at the same time."

## A *Star Is Born*

I myself am not immune to the pleasures of food and must confess also to having a weight problem. I am not fat, but I always have to watch what I'm eating. I was a skinny child. "Milly just doesn't eat," everyone said. My undernourished appearance was a constant source of embarrassment to my mother, who took it as a living reproach to her motherhood. I received a lot of attention from my mom, which I enjoyed. True, it was all negative — worries and sighs and fears for the future — but it was gratifying because I got so little approval from her. I settled for whatever I could get.

One day I discovered that when one food was mixed with another food on a plate, it was no longer the disgusting, unappetizing mess it had been when I wouldn't eat it at all until each kind was separated. Suddenly, the taste combination of mashed potatoes and lettuce became delicious. When I said I liked them together, I became a Star. A big fuss was made over me. "Milly likes something besides candy," they said, and every day there were mashed potatoes and lettuce. After four days in a row, I had had enough. "But I thought you liked it," my mom said. "I did," I said. "Yesterday."

Milk was another dinner table issue. To solidify my reputation, I refused to drink it. I was forced to sit at the table until I had finished the entire glass. "It's good for you," they said. I hated it. (I have never since touched milk, or vanilla ice cream or pudding or anything that tastes vaguely milky.) No longer a Star, my new reputation became that of a "finicky eater." They just couldn't fatten me up. I loved the attention. My eating problem was much discussed between my parents and even with their friends. I was Important.

When I was about twelve years old, I became overweight. Unhappy and self-conscious, I looked eighteen. My parents did not like the way I looked, and they made comments about my appetite. Once again, I had an eating problem, but on the other end of the scale. I had succeeded in doing what my mother wanted — I had gained weight — and no approval was forthcoming. The result was a confused self-image born of conflicting messages. I was good if I ate, and I was bad if I ate. I couldn't win.

As an adult I have spent much of my time fruitlessly trying to live up to two opposing ideas — eating more than I need to and staying thin. When I overeat I feel like a bad person. When I hold back, I feel deprived and punished.

## Vengeful Eating

Children catch on very quickly to the idea that overeating is an easy way to express their anger at their parents. Food is quiet and not perceived as being hostile. The fat child who gets disapproval from her parents for being fat can strike back very simply just by staying fat. It's a way of telling the world, "Everyone can see just by looking at me what bad parents you've been." The parents have no difficulty in getting the message, and neither does the rest of the world. The revenge continues even after the child is grown up, sometimes with a spouse or lover substituting for the parents.

## Mother and Daughter

A television talk show recently featured a group of famous movie actresses and their daughters. One of the actresses, a well-known international beauty, appeared with her sullen, obese twenty-year-old daughter. Asked about their relationship, the daughter replied in monosyllables. Viewers sensed that the last place in the world she wanted to be was there, with her mother. Her appearance was dramatic testimony to their relationship. Looking at her, we saw the story — the competition and the daughter's inability to compete, her rage, then giving up and taking refuge in food, food that would serve a double purpose: to get her out of the beauty-sex-men competition, and to revenge herself against her mother who prized beauty so highly and had a lump for a daughter. The rage also covered her fear that if she were thin and beautiful she would be a threat to her mother and lose whatever passes for love between them. Although she is grown up, part of her has remained a fat child. Her life is still dominated by her parent, if only in reaction to that parent. Her strongest drive is to hold onto her anger at whatever cost. The cost is self-destruction and an unrealized life.

Even if you feel you're a total adult, all grown up and in charge of your life, you can always blame your parents for the overeating you do today, *now*. Many people blame their parents for all the events that didn't work out in their lives. Often problems do originate early in life and are directly connected to the way your parents treated you. But that is really beside the point. Blaming your parents for your own shortcomings is merely a way of refusing responsibility for present behavior. It's taking the path of least resistance — not looking at yourself. Blaming your parents for your current eating record enables you to remain an innocent, victimized child.

•

Madeleine says, "I feel my mother hooked me on food. It's almost like being an addict. I was thin until I was about seven years old, and then I remember that she used to shove a little Good Humor Dixie cup in my face and say, 'Eat it, eat it, it's good for you.' She always did that when I was angry or crying or having a temper tantrum."

•

Gil, who started to overeat when he was in his twenties, says, "I had a terrible childhood. I never could do anything right. My mother was very strict, and my father always seemed to be angry at something. I figured it was me. I know they loved me, but they never really showed it. No matter what I did, I could never get their approval. When I grew up they wanted me to be happy, and that meant getting married. I've never married. I'm thirty-eight now, and it doesn't look as if I ever will. I'm so fat, no woman will look at me. It was the only way I could get back at them."

## Tug of War

When there is disagreement between parents, children feel both powerful and guilty — powerful because of all the attention they are getting, and guilty for causing an argument. If your parents had conflicts with each other over you, that too can become an excuse for overeating.

·

Jack, who was a fat child and still works at keeping his weight down, says, "When I was thirteen, I stopped eating so much. I lost weight and began to emerge from my fat cocoon and become a part of the world. It was mostly my own doing, with no help from my parents. My mother would say, 'Let him have it; don't worry about it; it's okay for him to eat another piece of cake.' My father would become enraged. He was concerned about me — all the hours I spent in my room and my being overweight — and I felt he kind of understood me. But he wouldn't go against her word. I, of course, reaped the benefit of having the cake, since she won."

·

Robert is 6 feet tall and weighs 245 pounds. "It was always my mother and me against my father in more ways than one. He'd come home from work and there would be wild fights about how the two of us had to lose weight and get all the junk food out of the house. When my father went to work, my mother and I would go out to the store and load up. We'd put one bag of chocolates in her lingerie drawer and another in one of my drawers. It was a game. When my father came home, we would sneak around the house and eat chocolate under his nose, thinking we were fooling him. It was their unhappiness with each other that got me into this overeating problem."

## Fat Families

There may well be a genetic predisposition to fat, as some researchers claim, but it is exacerbated by overeating. The eating habits of the parents are taught to the children.

•

Betty says, "I think one reason I'm still fat is that I don't feel independent and capable of making my own decisions. I have a husband to take care of me, and I still have my mother, who is also fat. I always wanted her to set an example for me as a woman, to be my role model. I'm very angry at her, and the anger is tied in with her weight problem. She just gets heavier and heavier. She doesn't take care of herself; she doesn't do anything for herself. She doesn't even seem to care, much less try. I'm afraid I'll end up like that."

## Soothing Foods

The fat child very often has been made to feel "different," as if there is something very wrong with him. Ridiculed and left out of the fun and games of other children, he is driven to food for consolation. Events conspire to feed the fatness. As an adult, he is likely to return to the same foods for help.

•

A sixty-four-year-old widow recently came to me for help. Her husband had died the month before. During the first period of her mourning, she was unable to eat anything at all, and then she started craving food that she had not eaten since she was a child. She went so far as to carry a sandwich in her purse, to make sure she had the right food with her at all times. Food was used to assuage her loneliness and pain.

## Ice Cream — The Primal Food

Ice cream is in a class by itself. It is *the* food to fall back on in times of stress. Almost a primal kind of food — smooth and creamy, nothing to chew, going down easily, effortlessly — ice cream is the reward most often given to a child who has performed well. Ice cream has happy associations — a birthday, a celebration, a family outing. Ice cream continues to be a soothing cure-all long after children have grown up.

•

Judy, who is forty-two, says, "I adore ice cream. I can't resist it. My mother had certain peculiar ideas about food. She thought it would make you sick to eat very cold food in the winter. We had lots of ice cream in the summer, but never in the winter. The winter I was six years old, I had my tonsils out. The doctor told my mother to give me soups and liquids, hot or cold; it didn't matter as long as they slid down easily. I remember sitting in bed, propped up with pillows, my throat achingly sore after the operation, hearing the doctor say, 'And ice cream. It's all right to give her plenty of ice cream.' It was as if ice cream was the reward for all that pain. I got a lot of soup, but I never saw any ice cream. My mother's fixation was stronger than the doctor's orders. From then on, ice cream became something very special for me. Whenever I had a headache — or any kind of ache — I knew that ice cream would make it feel better. I've used it to cure everything from indigestion to hangovers to loneliness."

## Switch

As a fat adult you are still taking care of hurts, angers, and frustrations with food. You remain a helpless, hungry infant. As such, you are unconsciously switching roles. To alleviate your discomfort — the craving, the emptiness, the deprivation — you feed yourself, thus becoming both the parent and the baby. You are the helpless, screaming infant, waiting uncertainly, wanting to be gratified *now;* and you are the parent, stuffing food into your mouth to stop the silent screaming. You are the parent, overfeeding yourself instead of giving yourself other good things, to make your life more satisfying. You are using food as the great pacifier, continuing the old primitive way of feeding.

## Early Messages

It is important to become aware of all these childhood patterns and messages. Too often we function without awareness, the way a chain smoker lights one cigarette after another without stopping to consider whether he really wants to smoke that cigarette. For compulsive overeaters, however, self-awareness generates a feeling of being punished: "When I'm on a diet, feeling better about myself, it's always like a little kid acting like a grownup. I can get away with it for so long, and then something happens. I become overwhelmed, and I have to be a little baby again. I go back to eating because being a grownup is too much work. I can't muster the energy. It's just too much responsibility to be attractive and look good. It's not real. The real me is a baby. I can only pretend for so long, then I have to go back to the real me. I begin to feel deprived, and I start feeding myself."

## Choose One

The choice is yours. You can choose to remain a child — or you can choose to control yourself and be an adult who takes self-responsibility. If you make a decision *not* to put one piece of food into your mouth, you have taken a big step toward taking charge of yourself. It may be that the next bite you'll eat as you have always eaten — but at least you will be aware that you have the power not to put the food into your mouth. Being aware, you are on your way to self-control.

# 5

# How Fat People Eat
—In Misery

*"Nobody gives me anything I want — I have to give it to myself."*

ALL OF US have painful feelings of anger, depression, loneliness, self-hatred, and we have our ways of coping with them. We try to forget them by watching television; we drown them in liquor or drugs; we lose them in sex or sleep — temporarily. None of these methods works for very long, and we find that at some point we have to confront the pain anyway.

Fat people most often try to hide the pain with food. It is convenient and available and a very quick painkiller. Food is your medication, and fat is the side effect. Feeling unhappy and wanting to eat are inextricably tied together; one triggers the other in a chain reaction. Often you're not sure of what you're feeling — a sign that something you don't want to handle is troubling you. (You know how quickly you feel good when you have something to feel good about.) So you have three factors to contend with: the pain, the extra pounds, and the self-recrimination for having allowed yourself to gain weight.

## What Do You Really Feel?

Do you find it hard to decide whether you're angry, depressed, sorry for yourself, or hungry?

Are you eating because you're lonely or are you eating because you're hungry?

Do you really want to polish off the leftovers in the refrigerator or do you *really* want to crawl into bed and cry?

•

Dorothy is angry at her ex-husband, who is lax in his child-support payments, not to mention alimony. When he says, "The check is in the mail," and it doesn't arrive, she becomes enraged and calls him. She knows he hasn't sent it. After she hangs up the phone, she feels she needs something to eat immediately. "I keep thinking that it goes back to being an infant. If you leave an infant alone, she will pick a balanced diet for herself. The way I eat now is something I learned since then. I want to go back to where I know what my body needs, where my body and mind will be one unit together. When I'm on a diet and feeling furious about something, I have to stop and think, '*Am I really hungry?* What do I really want? Do I want that cake or do I want to punch somebody?'"

## Who's Angry?

Many angry people are walking around who don't know that they're angry. They may elbow someone in the subway or kick and shove in a crowd — and never admit to angry feelings.

Most of us have been taught not to express anger or, if

we do, to try to be "nice" and do it in a "nice way." We believe there is something wrong with feeling anger and wanting to fight back when attacked. Releasing anger appropriately — the true, raging depths of it — not only is frightening to the person who releases it, but extremely threatening to others. If we allow ourselves to vent angry feelings, we are afraid of not being liked. Wanting to be liked is something of a national disease.

•

Connie, a therapist in a hospital, is afraid of her anger. She holds it back for a long time, then suddenly becomes furious with people. When Connie is occupied constructively with her work and nothing provokes her anger, she manages to lose weight consistently. When she is angry, she raids the refrigerator. When Connie became enraged at a co-worker for a minor infraction and lashed out at him, she no longer needed to eat. She justified her anger with, "In a crazy way, I felt good that I could express my anger rather than take it out on myself by overeating."

•

Elaine Kaufman, hostess to the endless parade of celebrities who dine nightly at her Upper East Side New York bistro, lost 205 pounds. When she was obese, she had a reputation for throwing people out of her restaurant at the slightest provocation, even if they were in the middle of their meals. The new Elaine is considerably mellowed. In a *New York Times* interview she said, "The hostility has dissipated a lot as I feel better about myself . . . I had a lot of hostility toward myself, and if I was antagonized it would come out . . . There's a lot of unhappiness in being fat because you're never confident. You are always insecure and angry with yourself, and your emotional thread is very thin."

## Cooled Out

If you are a "nice" fat person, the niceness is your way of not making waves. Expressing anger makes you stand out. It's bad enough to be overweight. But what happens to the anger? You teach yourself to disguise it in other unhappy feelings that are not as threatening to acknowledge to yourself:

|                |             |
|----------------|-------------|
| Helplessness   | Boredom     |
| Sadness        | Loneliness  |
| Resentment     | Self-hatred |
| Confusion      | Isolation   |
| Depression     | Numbness    |

These feelings are defenses against the dangers of genuine anger that you either don't know you are feeling or don't dare express.

•

Lila feels that her boss takes advantage of her — but she swallows his treatment of her without a word. "At ten minutes to five, my boss asked me to type three letters that had to go out that night. I told him I had a doctor's appointment at 5:45, but I felt guilty about telling him. I usually stay as long as he wants me to. After all, that's what I'm getting paid for — to do my job and be accommodating. Of course, last week I stayed till past seven o'clock three times. No, I didn't ask for overtime. I'm afraid to. I just didn't feel I had a right to tell him or to be angry. I felt absolutely rotten about myself. I went home, and instead of eating good food, I picked up a cake and ate the whole thing."

## Self-Pity

Twenty-year-old Katy says, "When I was in school last semester, I was doing a lot of work, feeling good about myself, and sticking to a diet. Now the semester is over and I
don't know what to do with myself. I've gained a lot of
weight. My life is unfocused. I should look for a job, but I'm
just sitting home and feeling depressed. All I do is eat."

## Anxious

Norma, a woman of forty who is 5 feet 4 inches and weighs
173 pounds, works as a secretary for a publishing company
and is thus not invited to editorial meetings. Norma thinks
the editors look down on her for not being their intellectual
equal and for being fat. She wonders what they talk about
at those meetings, and if some of what they say is about
her. She has suppressed these feelings so much that she
doesn't even know she has them. "I'm not aware of feeling
angry or even of feeling anxious. All I know is that I have
an urgent desire to chew or bite."

## Depression

Depression is a word that covers a lot of territory. There are
many different symptoms of depression, and people experience it in different ways. It may come over you suddenly,
and just as suddenly go away. It may linger for a long time
— weeks or months — and you feel you are inside a glass
jar, unable to touch anyone or anything. It may be caused
by tangible events — a broken love affair, a job loss, a death

— or its causes may be impossible to discover, and you just have to wait it out. As a rule, when people who are not preoccupied with food become depressed, they lose their appetite. They are unable to find solace in food; it becomes repulsive to them. Fat people handle their depression by feeding it, compulsively and nonselectively. They turn to what they know is always there for them, the one thing that offers comfort and company.

Jason, who is middle-aged, has had a weight problem all his life. He walks around in a semipermanent depression. Most of the time he is not aware he is depressed. "There are a lot of times when I want to call a woman or hang out with my friends, but I stay home, smoking grass and watching TV — and eating a lot of junk. I know the grass makes me hungry, but it also helps me not to feel. It's not that I don't want to lose weight. I just can't do anything good for myself right now. I'm being totally self-destructive, but I tell myself I'm being self-sufficient. I just feel too bad to face anything."

## Boredom

Other feelings — also painful, but easier to pin down — may be a cover for depression, as boredom is for a young mother in her late twenties. Sheila left an exciting job in public relations to stay home and take care of her first child. She wanted to be with her baby, especially during his early years, but she hates staying home. It's dull; it makes no claims on her mind. She feels shut out from the world. "I used to do a lot of traveling and a lot of running around with people. I felt free and I loved it. I love my baby too, but being with a baby all day is really boring. John is gone all day, and there's nothing going on. The only thing I like to do these days is eat. I'm always thinking about food. I can't wait to go to the supermarket. I'll often walk over to the refrigerator, and even though I'm not hungry, I eat. It passes the time."

## Hiding Unhappiness

Many of us consciously hide what we feel, whether it is anger, pain, or sadness. We don't want the outside world to know that we feel bad. Sitting on feelings becomes a deeply ingrained habit that generates enormous amounts of frustration. After a while, you no longer know *what* you feel, or if you feel anything at all.

•

Donald, who is 5 feet 8 inches and weighs 188 pounds, has a tense situation at home. "My wife makes me furious sometimes. She was complaining that I didn't do enough work around the house. The yard was full of leaves and needed raking, but I'm tired on Saturday after working all week. I want to relax. She called me fat and lazy. I felt guilty. If I could have gone to a gym and punched something out, I would have felt better, but I sneaked into the car and drove off to get something to eat. I turned it all on myself. I had an incredible need not to show anger. Just to do something."

## Loneliness

In her book *Bittersweet*, Terri Schultz describes loneliness as "a feeling of discontent and rejection. It is a sense of being helpless, trapped in a physical or emotional limbo. It comes when you feel threatened by being alone, when you feel something is missing. It is a desire for something outside yourself..."

Loneliness is a perfect excuse to eat or to go on a binge. You tell yourself you have a right to eat because nobody else is there to feed you or nurture you. The phone doesn't ring; that wonderful person you met last week hasn't called. Someone at the office gave a party and didn't invite you. You feel sorry for yourself. If no one else will give you what you want, you will give it to yourself.

•

Abe says, "Last weekend when my wife was away, I was hanging around the house, eating everything in sight. That's when it's really bad for me, when I'm alone and doing nothing. There's the sense that I'll feel better if I eat something."

•

Arnold says, "I look for reasons to eat, and I find reasons to feel bad. If I don't understand the way my girl friend has been behaving toward me, I'll think it's rejection — it's me, something she thinks is wrong with me. I always think it's my fault, but I don't know what 'it' is. I begin to feel like a helpless child; those old feelings come back, and I start to eat again. When I was little I ate because it drove my mother crazy and it punished me — it got to both of us."

•

Perhaps the most intensely painful feelings of loneliness well up during weekends and holidays. Raymond says, "I just don't think about food during the week when I'm busy and spending time with other people. I can even pass up potato chips then. But weekends and holidays are murder. Everyone in the world is having fun and feeling great and being with people, and I'm all alone. I can't even bring myself to go out in the park and see all those jolly groups. It makes me feel even more alone."

## Togetherness

Many people who are single, divorced, or who live alone often think that finding The Relationship they have always longed for will change their overeating habits.

•

Sally is one of those people. She found the man she wanted, married him, and had three children. After each child was born, she gained more weight. Her husband was busy with work and too tired after a long train ride to the suburbs to give her much in the way of companionship. He was even too tired to make love with her. Sally sublimates her pain by cooking gourmet meals for her family. It's an excuse for getting fat.

## Back to the Womb

At times, life just becomes overwhelming. There are too many demands, too many matters that have to be taken care of immediately. Altogether, life is unmanageable. A temporary retreat from pressure is not necessarily bad: once in a while everyone needs a little self-indulgence — staying in bed to read or watch TV. At such times, it is most difficult to resist the temptation to pamper ourselves with little treats to eat.

·

When she is in a funk, Isabel throws up her hands, blocks out the world, and takes to her bed. Wrapped in a quilt, safe and warm, she finds her secret escape in sleep. She doesn't even get dressed for two or three days at a time, doesn't answer her phone. "It's like having a mini–nervous breakdown. My room is an isolation chamber. I just stay in bed, feeling terrible, eating and sleeping. I cook a lot of starchy stuff, which is what really appeals to me when I feel this way. I feel warm and taken care of, and I start to think that maybe all the problems I can't cope with will just go away."

## Burned Out

Lorraine, who is twenty-four years old and always talking about losing weight, often hides from the world. Her hospital job, dealing with life and death on a daily basis, is extremely debilitating and takes a great deal out of her. She has to give of herself all the time. In the helping professions, there is a point at which one can no longer give. When that point is reached, the helpers need to be helped. This syndrome is called being "burned out." Lorraine is suffering from it. "Who is giving to me?" she asks. "What do I get for all I give?" There is no one around who will "give" to Lorraine. She has no close friends. "I'm feeling so fat and ugly," she says. "Last Wednesday I began to feel sick at work. Some pains and aches and the beginning of a cold. I stayed home in bed Thursday and Friday and watched TV all day and evening. I only got up from bed to get something to eat. By Thursday night I knew I wasn't sick, but I wanted to be. I took the phone off the hook. I just can't give anymore."

## Victim of Yourself

"I had not seen my friend Lorna for about a month," said Marie. "When I saw how thin she had become, I was jealous of her, and I felt angry at myself." Marie has been trying for years to lose about thirty pounds. Once she actually did it, but she has since put it all back on, and then some. Now she feels helpless, hopeless, and full of self-pity. "After seeing Lorna, I was determined to be thin too. But instead I went on a binge. I just can't seem to lose weight, and I feel lousy about myself."

•

Ruth is a woman with deep feelings of worthlessness. "When anyone gets angry with me, I start crying. It's very manipulative, I know. I want that person to feel guilty and sorry for what he did to me. Then I have a better excuse to eat. This wave of 'poor me' comes over me, and off I go. It makes me feel better about not doing anything."

•

Harry believes he has never been able to get what he deserves from life. Instead of going out and trying to get it, he eats. "I complain about being overweight. It's a tape in my head that I play for my friends so they won't bug me. I think I would like to take care of myself, that I'm worth it. But I'm a victim, and I always feel like a victim. Picked on. Everyone messes me over, and I'm such a wonderful person."

## Masochism

In the self-recrimination that follows each weight gain, many people descend to the depths of humiliation, paying money to be blasted with a sadistic message. A device called "Diet Conscience," which hooks up to the refrigerator, has been very popular. When the door is opened, the device, which has a nasty laugh, goes into action. "Are you eating again?" It cackles. "Shame on you! No wonder you look the way you do! Ha! Ha! Ha! You'll be sorry, fatty! Do yourself a favor; *shut the door!*"

When painful feelings are an invitation to eat, you become the victim of a necessity of life that has grown entirely too necessary. Fat is both the excuse for and expression of your unhappiness — and overeating prevents you from coming to grips with the causes of that unhappiness.

•

A small plump woman left my office last week after a particularly painful therapy session. As the tears dribbled down her face, she looked up at me and said, "The first thing I'm going to do when I leave here is get some glazed doughnuts." The following week she told me she had had to walk twenty blocks to find just the right kind, but she found them — and ate them.

# 6

# Feasts and Famines

*"When I'm on a diet, all I think about
is getting from one meal to the next. My
daily goal is to get to dinner."*

IN RECENT YEARS, eating has become one of our national
preoccupations. Time was when newspapers ran a few
recipes for housewives; now, entire sections, supported by
grocery advertisements, are devoted to buying and eating,
criticizing and rating food and restaurants. Thousands of
column-inches describe sumptuous dinners in sensual de-
tail, from appetizer to dessert.

New cookbooks encourage us to cook delectable dinners
at home. Every year, space in bookstores expands to accommodate cookbooks for the "in" cuisine and any lifestyle
— pastas or breads, Chinese or Mexican, one-dish meals for
singles, full-course dinners for couples.

A new industry has sprung up in service of the idea that
every American is his or her own gourmet with a machine
for each fashionable new food. Kitchen shops sell an endless
array of food processors, bread mixers, yogurt makers,
doughnut machines, corn poppers, pasta cutters — all the
accessories to prepare a complicated meal of the sort that
once required a chef, cooks, and assorted scullery maids.

Gourmet cooking has become part of the social-climbing, celebrity-imitating ethos of America. Eating itself is one of our more important social activities — picnics in summer, lunches with friends, business lunches, brunches, late suppers, sandwiches in bars. Our socializing is built around food.

Those who have no time or inclination to cook have a choice of thousands of fast-food chains, a constant invitation to gain weight. On every street corner and highway there are ice cream stores, doughnut stores, cookie stores, pizza stores, hot dog and soft drink stands. We nibble, gnaw, and nosh our way through the day, no longer able to see food simply as one part of a life that offers many other pleasures. In our snack culture, the pervasive emphasis is on quantity. More is better.

> All you can possibly eat
> A meal in itself
> Double whopper
> Big Mac
> 14-oz. steak
> Giant lobster
> Double-thick shake

We struggle constantly with the eating temptations around us, grabbing the quick fix to fill an empty space that has nothing at all to do with being hungry. In our country of plenty, why are we always stuffing ourselves with sugar and grease and fried dough?

A recent *New York* magazine survey asked thirty-seven public figures, "What is your secret vice?" Over half the answers involved eating. Gloria Vanderbilt said, "My secret vice is Godiva chocolates. I try to stay away from them, though. If I eat just one, there goes the box." Ed Koch, mayor of New York, confessed, "I'm a midnight snacker. When I have an anxiety attack, I go straight to the refrigerator." Liz Smith, syndicated gossip columnist, gets up in the middle of the night and eats "a whole bag of potato chips and a candy bar."

## Civilized Eating — The French

The French, too, have a national obsession with food, but theirs, as befits the national character, is more intellectual and philosophical. Articles in the French press tend to be self-critical and abstract, dealing with such subjects as, "Do we live to eat? Or do we eat to live?"

Unlike Americans, whose lunch is often a pit stop at a taco stand on the way to the tennis courts (California), a pizza eaten on the street (New York), or a box of fried chicken in the car (Tennessee), the French consider a meal an event. Food is served in courses, including wine, cheese, salad, and dessert, and portions are small by American standards. The French eat more slowly than we do, waiting and digesting between courses. There is a lasting satisfaction, both physical and aesthetic, in completing such a meal that the fast-food fix cannot provide. After eating it, there is little desire to keep nibbling until the next meal. Our manner of eating may have a lot to do with our fatness. Obesity does not seem to be a national problem in France as it is here.

## Eat/Don't Eat

At the same time as we are assaulted by food, we are told not to eat too much. Along with our preoccupation with food goes its opposite — a preoccupation with dieting. Eat, enjoy the abundance, become a gourmet, learn how to choose the right wine and cook thick creamy sauces and rich desserts — but don't gain any weight while you're ingesting three, four, or five thousand calories a day.

It is virtually impossible to pick up a magazine without finding at least one article on diet, nutrition, or exercise. Just about everyone has a theory about why you are fat and how to get rid of your excess weight. In addition to water, fat, carbohydrate, rice, protein, and liquid protein diets, there are group diets, behavior-modification programs, guided imagery (fantasizing feeling thin), fat-cell theory, fasting, starvation, jaw-wiring, intestinal bypass operation. *People* magazine recently conducted a reader survey on various topics of the day, including, "How many pounds would you like to lose?" From the answers, the magazine's editors calculated that the total national desired weight loss comes to nearly a million tons. To cater to this desire to be thin, diet books for new miracle transformations of our overweight bodies flood the market. The supermarket tabloids carry an "amazing new diet" every week. (Their most amazing feature is that people believe in them.)

The American appetite is worth over $200 billion a year. The food industry can't afford to let you stop eating. Instead, it developed the diet industry, which wants you to eat also, but pushes other kinds of foods — sugar-free, salt-free, fat-free, no-cal, dietetic, butterless, Weight Watchers, anything, as long as you eat. Everyone wants to make money out of your eating habits. Everyone wants you to buy food. How can you possibly resist? Especially when you need to eat just to survive.

What happens to all the people who buy the information and the diet food? Do they go on the diets? Do they lose weight? Vivian says, "I have been trying to diet for the past thirteen years. I went to the real Dr. Atkins, and I went to the guy who invented liquid protein. I've even had cow's-urine injections. I've tried everything, and here I am still fat."

You can resist the pressures if you understand exactly how you approach dieting and how that approach undermines you.

## Why Diets Don't Work

It doesn't matter what method you've chosen to lose weight or what diet you're on. All of them can work. They don't work because you don't really want to lose the weight. The comforts you derive from overeating are more important to you than losing the weight. To ensure that you don't lose those comforts, you either look for magic or you put responsibility for your weight loss elsewhere — on the doctor or the diet.

Both of these approaches guarantee failure.

## Magic

Many fat people believe that a force outside themselves will lose the weight for them. The idea of shedding pounds themselves — of determining to lose weight for no other reason than that they hate themselves fat — is an idea they avoid.

.

Jacob is forty-two years old and weighed 240 pounds when he was in the eighth grade. "People cop out their whole lives, trying to find short cuts. That's why self-help books and diet books get sold. I waited most of my life for the magic word to take me away, and I'm still fat. There's no magic trick. You just get in there and do it."

•

Ginny weighed 247 pounds. Getting down to 200 was her first goal. "I thought it would be easier after that. Two hundred was the magic number, and it took me so long to reach it. I thought losing the rest of the weight would be a cinch. It finally got through to me that I'm going to have to keep working as hard or harder to get the rest off."

## Jet-set Magic

In Paris, Dr. Robert Chung, diet doctor to the jet set, says, "Keep to food that can be eaten raw as well as cooked. In the primitive days before fire and ovens, our ancestors ate no bread or unnecessary carbohydrates. And they had no weight problems." Dr. Chung also dispenses exotic miracles. During the initial visit, he prescribes little pills of goats' ovaries, animal brains, and some strychnine. "These substances are harmless in small doses," he says. In addition, he prescribes a bottle or two of his own secret formula. His favorite exercise is disco dancing "because an evening with the Bee Gees can burn 900 calories."

Some of Dr. Chung's clients are international stars, people we would never dream have a weight problem, such as "wraithlike actress Marisa Berenson" and "superslim Pat Kennedy Lawford, who looks as though she subsists on roots and berries," and Princess Grace of Monaco. In an interview in *Réalités* magazine, Dr. Chung said he was often flown to the Persian Gulf to look after an oil-rich potentate's overweight harem. "Those poor women aren't very free to lead active healthy lives," he says. "After all, anybody would get fat sitting around all day at a gossip session or watching TV, nibbling at pastries or chocolates. Those ladies have a terrible sweet tooth, but they all want to be fashionable. How can you wear a St. Laurent if you're as big as Mae West?"

## Take Care of Me

Dr. Chung's fancy little pills, the diet books on the best-seller list, and your own diet doctor present the same approach to dieting — the search for an authority, for someone to assume responsibility for your fat. Instead of using the diet, the pill, the injection, the exercise machine as tools, you expect them to lose the weight for you. There's nothing wrong with any of these devices if they work. What *is* wrong is that you use them as a crutch — which puts you in the position of being dependent, like a child. Like a child, you feel you have no control over your life. Adults try to handle their problems; children need to have someone more powerful check on them and give them direction.

When you want to lose weight, you think: "I can't do it by myself. I've tried and it's no good." You go to a diet doctor who says: "This is what you are to eat — so many calories per day. These for lunch, these for dinner, no substitutions. Do what I tell you like a good patient, and you will take off so many pounds."

By supervising your food intake, diet doctors become parents to you. They know more than you do; they have the final word. You have a childlike faith that although the doctor is strict, he or she will take good care of you.

But soon you begin to think the doctor is too easy on you.

He or she isn't paying that much attention to you any-more; the nurse is weighing you and evaluating your progress. You really want a controlling parent, and you're not getting one. The doctor is telling you that *you* have to take care of your weight; it's your responsibility. You stop going to the doctor. And then you can say, "I went to a doctor, but it didn't work."

If you're not in charge, the failure is not your fault. The doctor is in charge — it's the doctor's fault. As long as you continue to lose weight, the doctor is good, someone you can rave about to your friends. As soon as you stop losing or start gaining, the doctor loses ability or becomes a quack. You get off scot-free — no failure or blame attaches to you for not losing weight, and you can go back to eating every-thing you want again. You win — but you're still fat.

## Sexism

Most diet doctors are men, and most of their patients are women. In continuing to look to men for guidance, as parental and medical authorities, women are encouraged to remain dependent on them and to look for authorities out-side themselves.

Men, on the other hand, have a different problem. An obese male patient who has never been on a diet told me, "Men don't diet as much because men don't admit to any-thing. They won't admit to any frailties; they won't admit to any failures. It's a macho thing. Men don't want to go in groups and tell a lot of women that they're fat. I know men who diet, but they do it secretly and quietly and very much on their own. It doesn't become a big issue, and they don't tell people about it."

## Pills and Injections

As authorities, doctors can tell you to do something that you know doesn't feel right or even make sense, and you will do it. For example, most diet drugs are amphetamine based. They are highs, dangerous and addictive — and "speed" kills. But the doctor tells you to take them and to come back next week for more. The doctor is the person who is going to cure you of being overweight, the person who will approve of you when you lose weight. You swallow your questions along with the pills, figuring that your weight loss will more than compensate for the danger.

Many people who went the drug and injection route and lost weight feel negatively about the experience of pill dependency. But they are still looking for miracles.

•

Monica, who is obese, ran into an old friend who had lost seventy pounds on appetite depressants and injections. "On principle, I really hate shots and pills. But right away I got excited — this could be the doctor who'll do it for me. He'll take the responsibility. Maybe it's worth it."

## One of the Crowd

Whether you buy a diet book, visit a doctor, or concoct your own regimen, being on a diet does something very important for you if you are fat. It transforms you from an outsider to an insider. Since everyone else is on a diet, at last you "belong." You like the feeling of telling people what diet you're on, of carrying your special lunch to work — a container of yogurt, a can of tuna, an apple — for everyone to know how good you are, how conscientious. You have a subject for conversation, a subject that everyone wants to talk about; you are no longer "different." You hear wonderful stories of how people have lost fourteen pounds in two weeks, and you feel particularly motivated to stay on your diet. Everyone else is losing weight, and you will too.

## Discouragement

It's the fifth day of the diet and you weigh yourself as usual. You haven't lost any weight since yesterday. Worse, you've gained a pound or two. What went wrong? Whatever it was, you tell yourself that the diet just didn't work for you. Maybe there's something wrong with you? You feel deprived, empty. You go on a little binge to cheer yourself up, and pretty soon you've gained back all the weight you lost. You allow the binge to be fatal to the diet.

As soon as you deviate from the rules — and a dieter almost inevitably cheats — you feel guilty, like a bad child. An adult could shrug it off, treat it as a minor lapse, and go back on the diet. But you don't. You treat it as if it were the end of the world. You're too ashamed to return to your doctor. You revert to your old ways. You give up.

## Groupies

The most successful dieting methods I have heard about are those of Weight Watchers and Overeaters Anonymous, though no membership numbers are available and neither organization does followup studies. Their success hinges on the sharing of painful feelings. The worst part of dieting is the loneliness and isolation, feeling like a freak, believing that other people can eat normally and eat everything.

At a meeting you are no longer the lone freak. Other people in various stages of fatness or thinness are there; the thin people, who have already lost weight, offer encouragement; the fat people (you think) are fatter than you are. Rituals help — the supportive phone calls from Overeaters Anonymous sponsors, the weighing of the foods on the little scale at Weight Watchers.

•

Barry, a thirty-four-year-old advertising executive, says, "I lost thirty-one pounds using the Weight Watchers program, which is not a strict diet. In six weeks I went from 178 to 147. I didn't exercise a bit during that time. If your calorie intake is less, it's just mathematics that you are going to lose weight. I'm eating more now than I was when I was heavy, but I eat differently. I eat a protein breakfast instead of a corn muffin. It's half the calories. I've changed my attitude."

•

Another Weight Watcher says, "When I find that I have gained about ten pounds, I go back to the meetings. By myself, I just don't take as much care with my diet. The group helps motivate me."

•

Not everyone who loses weight keeps it off. Enthusiasm for the new experience wears off, and you slip back to your fat eating habits. Whether you lose weight or not, you never stop being compulsive about food. Indeed, the Overeaters Anonymous philosophy is that if you're a compulsive overeater you have to learn to be a compulsive noneater.

•

Douglas is a compulsive overeater. He used to be obese, but he lost over 170 pounds and has kept it off for more than ten years. "Someone asked me why I'm so compulsive about eating, and I said, 'Why do I have to have a reason? Why can't I just be hungry?' I'm hungry now, and you know what I just ate? Two scrambled eggs, three pieces of sausage, a toasted buttered bagel, and two cups of coffee." Food still controls Douglas's life. Not only does he think about nothing but eating, he owns a chain of restaurants. He has built his life around food and dieting. "I'm a foodaholic. I'm obsessed with food. I love food, and I think food is happiness. It's everything good in the whole world."

•

Compulsive overeating is often thought of as an addiction. In many ways it is. Just as former alcoholics and drug addicts have to be careful for the rest of their lives, so do food addicts. But there are differences. Drug and alcohol victims often become aware of an acute life-threatening element in their addiction. Obese people usually do not perceive themselves as vulnerable to their food in that particular way. In spite of medical warnings that obesity contributes to major illnesses, fear does not seem to be an important factor in losing weight. (The same is true for smokers and highway speedsters.) After all, food is necessary for survival. How bad can it be? And, there are differing medical opinions as to how much of a health threat overeating actually poses. Fat people (compulsive overeaters or not) who aren't absolutely sure they want to take the weight off, will always manage to find a way to keep it on. For them, dependence on doctors and diets and pills is one of the best ways to stay fat.

# 7

# How Fat People Fool Themselves into Remaining Fat

*"Don't tell me anything I don't want to hear."*

WHEN YOU THINK about where the responsibility lies for your weight problem, you know perfectly well that it lies with you. *But* — when you think about the reasons why you overeat and the excuses you make for yourself, the responsibility somehow shifts to other people's behavior toward you. Their actions often make the difference between whether you will eat or not.

Think of all those fast trips to the refrigerator, to the cabinet where the potato chips are kept. Think how often you make them when you're angry, saying to yourself, "I'll show her." You want to punish someone, to get back at someone who may have criticized you or disapproved of you or just said the wrong thing. You couldn't express your anger then and there, but you had to get back at that person somehow.

Eleanor says, "When my boy friend tells me I'm getting chunky, or worse, that he isn't attracted to me when I'm chunky, I really shove the food into my mouth."

•

Sometimes the opposite happens. There are all the times you're feeling good and you make the same trips to the refrigerator — only now it's a celebration; you're rewarding yourself because something nice happened.

•

Diana says, "Sometimes when I diet for a few days and lose a few pounds, somebody will notice and say to me, 'You look terrific. You lost some weight.' If I could only hold onto that it would be wonderful, but I pat myself on the head and start stuffing my face."

•

You are caught in the punishment-and-reward cycle. Either way, you lose. By punishing others, you are also punishing yourself. By rewarding yourself, you are also punishing yourself. In both cases, you are depending on something outside yourself to regulate the amount of food you take in. You are not taking responsibility for your overeating.

Such lack of control is not easy to admit. All of us would like to see ourselves as competent and rational people who know what we are doing and why we are doing it at all times. But we are not all competent and rational — certainly not all the time — and in order to maintain that self-image, we have to deceive ourselves in various ways.

## *Tricking Yourself — Thinking Thin and Acting Fat*

Fat people rationalize choosing to stay fat. When the moment of truth comes, self-discipline and will power dribble away. Self-control vanishes.

Confronted with a decision, you know and you prefer not to know that you have to lose weight. You don't want to know because you don't want to go through the ordeal, or change your life. Instead, you fool yourself through a series of excuses, such as disbelief, procrastination, fear of the unknown, dependency. Here are some common tricks that allow you to deny the fact that you are fat:

1. Since you lost a little weight, you think you can reward yourself with a little binge because (a) you feel lonely; (b) she didn't call; (c) the kids are driving you crazy; (d) you feel thin.

2. Three-quarters of a quart of ice cream is sitting in the freezer. You tell yourself, "Well, just this once." You eat three spoonfuls and can't leave the rest. You think the ice cream won't make that much difference to your diet.

3. You have been dieting for a week and have lost only three pounds. There must be something very wrong. You were so careful. Why didn't you lose more than three? Well, you think, I'm not meant to lose weight. I'll give it up.

4. Now that you have lost some weight, you think you can eat normally. What is normally? Do you know?

5. You think that thin people don't have to be that careful. Now that you feel you are thin, you stop being careful.

6. You spent a lot of money to join a gym, but somehow, you always have a reason not to go there.

7. After three months of dieting, having lost a considerable amount of weight, you feel entitled to eat all the goodies you missed. When you get on the scale and see that you are five pounds heavier, you don't believe you've actually put on that weight. How can that be? Aren't you a thin person now?

## No Present

We all do it. We think in terms of yesterday and tomorrow, as if there were no today, or as if the things we are doing today are not important. We live in the past or the future — a past made rosy by memory; a future glorified by unreal expectations. It is a universal trait, and we all do it *some* of the time. If you are fat, you think that way *most* of the time — especially when your thoughts turn to losing weight. It's so easy to live through a wonderful past and a remarkable future that may never arrive. Today is just a hyphen, a link between the real periods of your life.

Usually, you are not aware that you are doing it.

Not thinking about today is a technique to avoid facing the problem of *now* — the problem of losing weight.

## The Past — The Memory of Thin

So many statements and references begin with the phrase, "When I was thin." You speak nostalgically of it, as a time forever past, a time of happiness that will never come again. "In the spring, when I was thin, I was feeling like a whole person. I had the image of myself as someone on a pogo stick or a trampoline, everything bouncing and moving. I felt good about myself physically and emotionally."

## The Future — Postponing Your Life

"I love to go to the beach and get a dark tan — I look terrific with a tan — but I've been so overweight during the last few years. I got rid of my bathing suits a long time ago, and now I don't ever go to the beach. I'm not only embarrassed about my pot belly, but about my white pasty skin. There are two marks against me."

•

"I say I'm not going to do a particular thing until I lose weight. I'm not even going to try. If I want to get picked up in a bar, say, I'm not even going to go to a bar until I lose that weight. Everything depends on losing weight. Everything seems not so immediate. You don't have to do it today. You don't have to do *anything* today."

## Too Big or Too Small

Many fat people fool themselves by buying clothes that are too small and will hang in the closet "until I lose the weight." Others buy clothes that are too big so that they can think about having them taken in — another way of believing they are really losing weight.

•

"Yesterday, before I went to a job interview, I put on my gray skirt that's too big in the waist," said Selma, not mentioning that she bought it a size too big.

•

"I don't want to buy clothes that fit," said Sandy, "because then I'd have to face the fact that I'm a size 36 and that's too painful."

## Pounds to Go

When you're thinking in terms of having to lose fifty or a hundred pounds, it becomes frightening and unmanageable. How can you sentence yourself to diet and deprivation for an interminable length of time? You can't think of it as a little bit every day, a gradual melting-off process. All you see is that big number looming up ahead of you in the future. To avoid the diet, you use the device of becoming overwhelmed by the numbers. "I weigh over 200 pounds and I think, 'My God, look at all the weight I've got to lose.' I can't possibly do it."

## The Numbers Game

"Tomorrow I will go on a diet," you say, knowing that tomorrow will never come. "In my mind I used to have an ideal weight that I wanted to reach. I would lose some weight, and then I would gain it back before I hit the magic number. It was a game I played against myself so that I would always lose. I haven't been on a scale in a long, long time."

## Blaming Others

No matter what kind of attention you get from other people about your weight, it never seems to be the right kind. When other people criticize you about your weight, it means they don't love you. On the other hand, when they *don't* criticize you, it means they don't care about you. They don't notice you; they don't see *you*. Nothing they can say or do is right. The blame is placed outside yourself, never on you, and you continue to feel like the baby no one wanted to take care of.

There are no winners in this secret baby battle you wage against those who care about you. Friends don't even know that you are waging a war. Instead of being openly angry at the comments made about your weight, you use the stifled anger against yourself — you eat it.

It's very convenient.

## It's All Your Fault

Vicky, a twenty-five-year-old woman who is 5 feet 2 inches and weighs 140 pounds, says: "I ask my boy friend why he doesn't tell me I'm getting fat, and he says that when he does I scream and yell at him. He can't have sex with me for two weeks because I'm so angry with him. Well, sure, I don't feel attractive or sexy when I hear things like that. And you know how it ends? I say to him in my head that he doesn't love me and I'm going to eat more, and it's all his fault."

•

Alexandra is confused about the way she looks. Her confusion is brought on by a combination of desire and delusion — the desire to be what someone else wants her to be and the delusion that that image of herself is what she really is. "I was living with a man who likes plump women. He kept saying that he could feel my bones and that I needed to put on weight. I believed him. I thought I was too thin, even though I was twenty pounds overweight. If he thought I was attractive, then I was. I was really using it as an excuse to eat as much as he did. He was very skinny. When we broke up, I couldn't eat anything. I lost a great deal of weight without even trying."

•

Many people don't actually come straight out and put the burden on others for their overeating but approach it in a roundabout way: If other people don't stay with you and occupy your time, you'll have to resort to food.

•

"I had a really nice weekend," Evelyn said. "I went to a party, met a terrific guy, and we spent the whole weekend together. I wasn't hungry the whole time. On Sunday when he was getting ready to leave, I started getting hungry again. When he left I started to think that maybe he wasn't so terrific after all. I began feeling fat and unattractive, and I went to the refrigerator."

## Fat Ages

Not only is that feeling of neglect a very sensitive area for you and those around you, but the question of age may crop up to complicate matters. Fat people generally look older than they are.

•

Lois says, "When my husband tells me I'm gaining weight and that I look matronly, it really hurts. But when his back is turned, I eat. I pull everything out of my secret hiding places that no one knows about. It's very comfortable to be at home and eat the food that I keep for emergencies. Sometimes I offer some of it to my husband, and then he can't yell at me for having it in the house."

## "If You Can't Do It for Yourself, Do It for Me"

How many times have you heard that plea from your family or lover? And how many times has it antagonized you? They're trying to help, but you know perfectly well that you can't and won't lose weight for anyone else. You have to do it for you. What are they really trying to do? Are they really trying to control you?

You need so much reinforcement from others; you're dependent on outside approval; yet you antagonize people with your weight and your constant eating. Your response is such that you won't get the reinforcement. "You see?" you convey to them. "You're not helping me. You're just making it worse." This attitude is almost bound to engender guilt or remorse in them, and that helps you to go on eating.

•

Roz is a woman whose weight has gone up or down according to the amount of control she exercises over her men. "My current boy friend never says anything when I put on weight. He says that I get an attitude, a look on my face that puts him off completely, and I seem to get fatter. He's right. I get so mad at him, I just eat — and that makes me madder."

•

Patty says, "When I was going with Peter, we would argue a lot about how heavy I was, and he would walk out. The minute he split, I would lose weight. I realized that I'd have to meet new guys and look good and do my whole number. Peter and I broke up three times, and each time I'd lose weight. Then we would get back together and I would just put it on again. That should have told me something."

## Sexual Revenge

"I'm gonna show him. I'm gonna be so fat he'll have a real reason to reject me." Joanna is angry at George, who usually calls on Monday night. He didn't call last Monday night, and he didn't call for three Monday nights before that. That's a long time for Joanna to be getting back at him. She has been going on a binge every Monday night for three weeks so she can say to herself that George is rejecting her only because she has put on so much weight. George, of course, doesn't know, nor does he even care.

## Dependency

When you feel you're being taken care of, you begin to need the person who is taking care of you and to expect a certain continuity. You relax in the knowledge that someone is there for you. When the care is removed — when a spouse or a lover leaves, or a parent dies — the sense of loss is more acute because you suddenly have to look after yourself. For many people, it is frightening or angering. Instead of rising to the challenge of independence, they take refuge in food.

.

"When Marie left, the whole house fell apart. She took care of everything — the housekeeping, the bills, the repairs — and I can't seem to do anything by myself. The place is a mess, and I've been on one long binge."

.

Bill, who is thirty-two, 5 feet 11 inches, and weighs 220 pounds, has stopped trying. "I lost forty-five pounds when I fell in love. I wanted to look good for Harriet. When the romance was over, I put all the weight back on again. Now I can barely move to do any exercise. I used to love to exercise. I don't feel I have anything else to look forward to in my life but meals. I've kind of given up the chase and let myself get more and more self-indulgent. It's not worth the trouble, going after women."

•

Annabelle is married and very dependent on her husband. "If he should leave, I don't know what I would do. In some way, I'm putting a wall around myself. I don't feel attractive when I'm fat. I know I can be more attractive, but I'm not sure how other people would respond to me. My husband accepts me as I am, even though he's not happy with my fatness."

## I Don't Want to Grow Up

Rachel clerks in her father's store. It is a job that is beneath her capacities and she doesn't like it much, but it's safe and secure, and her father takes care of her. Every so often Rachel decides that she can't stand it and that she's going to find a better job. She makes up her mind that she is going to lose weight — but somehow she never does. She doesn't do anything about qualifying for another job either. Rachel wants to remain a child and be taken care of by an uncritical parent. Going out on her own means becoming independent.

## Fear of Losing Weight

To average people who worry about losing five or ten pounds, it seems incomprehensible that there should be any fear connected with losing weight. They have lost the weight before, and they can do it again. It is merely a question of being less self-indulgent, of sacrificing a few starches and sweets. But for those who have been conspicuously overweight for a very long time, it is another story. They have become adjusted to their bodies. They're comfortable with a certain way of eating, and thus a way of life. The idea of changing all that can be terrifying. They think there will be new ways to behave, that the old familiar ways will no longer do. They are used to a way of life that may have its unpleasant aspects, but the very familiarity of it is consoling, easy to handle.

Change means becoming a whole new person. What is it like to be a thin person? You feel like an immigrant to a country whose culture you know very little about. Can I speak the language? Can I adjust to the mores and the laws of the nation? How should I handle myself? All these unknowns can be so frightening that many times you decide against losing the weight.

·

Maxine says, "A few years ago I was heavy, and I wanted to lose weight. I stopped drinking and stopped smoking grass, and I had a very easy time. But now I just haven't got any conviction about losing weight. I don't have any motivation. I also have a real gloomy feeling that as I get older, it's harder to do anything at all."

·

After she lost weight Cecile became a desirable and attractive woman — but she was afraid to behave that way. She was afraid of sex. Her thin body was at odds with the way she thought and felt. She has become fat again. She asks, "Was my life really better than it is now? If I become thin again, will I be disappointed?"

## I Still Want to Be Different

Myra works with a close-knit group of people who see each other outside of work. Myra, the fat one, has her own role to play in the group, and is worried that she would have to take on a new role if she were to lose weight. "We're all about the same age, and there's a lot of competition — for clothes, dates, sports, friendships. If I lost weight, I wouldn't stand out as the one who is overweight. I might be less shy and relate to people more — I don't know. Now, mostly I don't get involved; I sort of stay by myself. Since I had my hair cut, I've had three people say, 'Oh, you cut your hair, it looks great. I really like that style. Now, if you'd lose weight . . .' If I lost weight I would have to relate to friends in a different way, feel like one of them, feel equal instead of different. I don't think I would even know how to do that. If I were thin, I'd have to be in the competition, and I'm afraid of that."

•

Faith, who is twenty-six years old and weighs over 170 pounds, is ambivalent. Although she doesn't date, she would like to; although she wants to be attractive, she is frightened of what it might bring. Faith can go on telling herself that the men she knows have a good reason for not asking her out. They don't find her attractive because of her weight. Suppose she didn't have the weight and they still didn't ask her out? How terrible she would feel! That would be another reason to put all those pounds back on again.

## *Identities*

For many fat people, being noticed obese is better than being ignored thin. "When you're overweight you have a lot more presence," said Ben, who is 5 feet 10 inches and weighs over 250 pounds. "If you lose the weight, then you won't have any substance to you. You have an identity. It's also a way of controlling the way people respond to you."

•

Gilbert, who is twenty-nine years old and 6 feet 2 inches, lost 110 pounds — and found that he had lost his identity along with the weight. "I was the classic jolly fat person. I used to make fat jokes about myself. It took away the pain. It was a bad identity, but it was an identity. I played on people's sympathy. Now that I'm thin, I'm just like anyone else. No one looks at me. I was paid attention to as a fat person — at parties, I had standard routines. I would put up a wall and do my routines, on and on, making fun of myself. It was self-flagellation. I would think, deep down, that people must like me because I could deal with my fatness. I never stopped to analyze it. I fooled myself. Now I don't go to parties as often. I get bored. Why go to a party if you can't eat or drink? If you're the only sober one? . . . I used to drink a case of beer a day. Since I dropped the routines, it's tough to deal with social situations. People don't expect too much of you when you're fat, so you don't have to deal with feelings. Now, I'm a changed person. I got contact lenses and had my hair frizzed . . . It's very depressing to have to be normal. I still want to be funny. I wanted to be a standup comic. People tell me I'm not as funny as I used to be. I don't know what I am."

## Power

Suzanne, a college professor who weighs over 300 pounds, told me she was desperate to lose weight. She hated everything about being fat and worried constantly about it. She changed her bed linens every other day; she groomed herself carefully, bathing twice a day, afraid that she might smell. She ate practically nothing — she *swore* that all she had for lunch was half a sandwich and a sip of Coke — and couldn't understand why the weight wasn't coming off. I referred her to an endocrinologist, thinking she might have a gland problem. Then the truth emerged. In spite of all its drawbacks, the fat made her feel powerful. When she walked into a room people paid attention to her and, in some cases, deferred to her. It was her personality that was so powerful, not her fat, but she was afraid she would lose that quality if she lost the weight.

## Where Is the Payoff?

One of the great mysteries about people who have managed to lose a lot of weight is why and how they put it back on again. The answer is not very difficult to find. When you have gone to the trouble of losing 50 or 150 pounds only to realize that life is not as wonderful as you expected it to be, being thin no longer seems worth the effort. You still have all the problems you always had — the problems that made you overeat to begin with.

Suddenly you think, so what if I'm thin? Nothing marvelous is happening. You're afraid to go out and buy new clothes, even though you had planned to reward yourself with them. You really aren't sure you're going to keep the weight off. The trouble is, you're not getting the instant gratification that overeating used to give you. You feel sad. What was the point of losing all that weight? What are you getting for it? You begin to slip back into your old ways. It's so much easier to gain the weight back than it was to lose it.

·

Cliff had a fantasy of being surrounded by women, having them fall all over him in their eagerness to be with him. His telephone would ring all the time, he thought; he would be a man-about-town. When he lost weight, it didn't happen — and he gained it back.

·

Peggy has recently lost thirty-seven pounds and looks fine — but the rest of her life is a disappointment. "I'm finding that my having lost weight is a point of tension between me and one of the other women I live with. She'd been away for a couple of months and hadn't seen me since I lost weight, and she keeps making little digs and talking about diets and how I'll grab all the men. I'm not grabbing any men. Being thin is a way to be accepted, but I'm also afraid that people are going to reject me if I look happy." Peggy keeps wondering about the rewards she was supposed to get — the popularity, the affairs, the men clamoring for dates. She is not even getting approval from her roommate.

## Justifications

If you are like many fat people, you have set up a pattern of protecting yourself from the truth — a pattern of avoidance. The truth is that you need to lose weight. Facing the truth means making a decision to do something about it — and that is painful.

•

Mitchell, who is obese, says, "I never wanted to admit to myself before that I was fat. It was too threatening. It always had to be put to me as a matter of: You don't *have* to lose weight, but it would be nice if you did. If I admitted to myself that I was fat, then I would *have* to lose weight, and I wasn't ready to accept that."

•

To protect yourself from the truth, you come up with justifications for remaining fat. Do you recognize any of the people below?

*The Accordion.* You have lost weight many times in your life, but each time you have gained it back. When you are criticized, you quickly point out that you *do* have the ability to diet — but the weight always comes back. So why bother? After all these years, even you have come to believe it.

*The Entitled.* You lose weight and you look good, and then you promptly reward yourself with an eating binge. You can see and feel the weight creeping back on, but you justify yourself to others by saying you deserve the food for a job well done. What you are really telling your critics is that you "deserve" to be fat.

*The Stabilizer.* You have lost seventeen of the forty pounds you need to lose. But you just can't face the other twenty-three pounds. It's too overwhelming. So you tell yourself how much better you look and feel, and that is good enough. When asked about your weight, you cheerfully announce that you have stabilized, whatever that means.

*The Procrastinator.* You have too many other problems right now. You tell people, "I have to get my head together (or my life together) first." You believe your weight problem is caused by other emotional difficulties, and you're right — but you use them as an excuse for postponing your most obvious problem, your obesity. You will take care of it later.

*The Success.* You don't like to fail, and you've always failed at losing weight. So you stop trying. Now you're a success — you're never going to try again. You know that you *could* have been a success had you put your mind to it.

*The I-Know-Where-I-Stand.* You are afraid to lose weight. Being thin will give you a brand-new life — and a set of brand-new problems. You hate being fat, but you've learned how to cope with fat-person problems. You've had wonderful fantasies about what life as a thin person would be like — but what if you lost all that weight and your life didn't change? Suppose it got worse? Right now, you know where you stand, and you question whether being thin is worth the sacrifice and the deprivation of being on a diet. To become thin would be like switching professions in midlife.

You can probably add one or two justifications of your own that you use as preventive medicine to keep yourself fat and round. Why not make a list of them? You might learn some interesting things about yourself — things you hadn't wanted to confront before.

# 8

# How Fat People Love
# —In Anxiety

*"When I'm about to make love, I un-
dress in the dark. I don't want anyone
to see me naked."*

FAT PEOPLE often use sex as a test. Bed is where the danger is greatest of having the most intimate secrets revealed.
If you are attractive in bed despite your self-hatred, you
have found another way of saying you don't have to lose
weight. You can be loved just the way you are.

•

Howard, who has always been fat and weighs over 240
pounds, has never been able to find a woman who wanted
to go to bed with him. Finally, in desperation, he engaged
a prostitute to spend an afternoon and evening with him.
She made him feel comfortable, loved, and happy. After
such a wonderful experience (forgetting that he paid for
it), he is more than ever unable to see why he needs to
lose weight. If this woman could love him, then so can
other women. He says, "If I could only find a woman like
that to live with, I could be happy and achieve something
in my life."

## Testing, One, Two . . .

Mariko, who is about fifteen pounds overweight, has a great deal of self-confidence in business, but manages to turn almost every encounter with a man into a bad experience for herself. She complains that she can't find a boy friend and develop even a "meaningless" relationship. Mariko makes sure that none of her relationships develop. Recently, she hit it off with a man at a friend's beach house, but the next morning he was cool and distant. "He said he had to get back to the city. He didn't even ask for my phone number. The minute he left, I headed for the refrigerator. I needed something right away. I figured my body turned him off."

When Mariko meets a new man, she unconsciously sets up a test for him: "If you make me feel attractive and wanted, I will be a sex object for you; I'll do anything you want." After the conquest is made, she begins to look for signs of rejection: his desire for another drink when she is impatient to get to bed, his taking too long in the bathroom, his not cuddling her enough. Everything is grist for her mill. She dissects every moment, and always to her own disadvantage. Mariko perceives lovemaking as a way to make herself feel better about herself. She doesn't think in terms of mutuality, or that the man might have insecurities too. Immediate gratification is her goal.

## Secrecy Versus Openness

Even in the 1980s, sex is still a subject not always easy for people to discuss. Too many battle-scarred veterans of the sexual revolution feel that the victory was not theirs. For them, the new openness about sex is more of a problem than the old secrecy. Secrecy at least was safe. Now that the experts have told them what they should be experiencing, they are even more reluctant to talk about sexual problems than they were before the revolution. There is no escaping the fact that their sex lives do not bear scrutiny under the new standards of ecstatic multiorgasms and no hangups. It has become too embarrassing to admit that the whole business may be causing you more anxiety than it's worth. The new openness is twice as inhibiting for fat people.

Secretly, you feel ashamed of your body. Confronted on every side with slim, perfect bodies in the media, you are constantly reminded of your physical inadequacies. Although there is no way for *anyone* to measure up, it is impossible for an overweight person even to approach such a vision.

·

Midge, who is a few pounds overweight (although she is the only one who would notice it), was telling me about her boy friend's interest in trying group sex. "I told him I wasn't into group sex," she said, "but the truth is that I think my body is too lumpy. I might consider doing it if I weighed two pounds. You know what I mean — not an ounce of fat. But not the way I look now."

## Body Image

Fat people very often ruin sex for themselves by refusing to allow themselves to enjoy it. They worry about the effect of fat on performance, and they are preoccupied with what their own body looks like — the flab and sag and cellulite, the lumps and bumps and stretch marks, and the just plain fat. They are all wrapped up in themselves. Sexuality, the ability to let go, is never given a chance. Most people don't realize that the greatest enemy of their sexuality is *not* their fat body. The real enemy is self-involvement. The all-important question — *How does the other person feel?* — is rarely on the fat person's mind. What are the other person's needs, desires? Is it possible that he or she too suffers from insecurities about sex?

Instead of concentrating on having a good time, fat people are absorbed in self-doubt. Before, during, and after sex, one or more of the following thoughts run through their minds:

1. I wish I could turn out the light.

2. How can I hide the fat if I have to undress in front of him (her)?

3. Maybe she (he) won't notice the stretch marks and bulges.

4. Why did I eat all that spaghetti and ice cream last night? I just know every bit of it shows.

5. I hope I can get an erection fast. My penis looks so small and limp under my stomach.

6. My breasts are so huge. Maybe he likes big-chested women.

7. He told me he likes women who have big asses. Why hasn't he called?

8. That man at the next table is looking at me. He must be interested in my girl friend, not me. Or maybe he's wondering why I'm so fat.

The premise underlying these uncertainties is that no one wants to sleep with a fat person, that fat is too repulsive for anyone to want to get close to. The reality is sometimes different.

## Do Men Really Like Fat Women?

Most men, it is thought, subscribe to the *Playboy* magazine ideal of female beauty. That an ordinary man who is not overweight — who might even be thin — would prefer a fat woman comes as something of a surprise to most people. There are many such men. One of them told me that when he is in bed with a thin woman he has to fantasize a fat woman in order to climax. Another explained his "strange taste" for fat women by saying he liked to think they were gaining weight just for him. This made him feel powerful.

These men are embarrassed by and ambiguous about their sexual preference. On the one hand, they want to be with a fat woman; on the other, they wonder what the outside world will think of them.

In a survey of men in *Big Beautiful Woman,* writer Maggy King asked, "Do you like big women?" Some of the replies:

A BUS DRIVER: I'd rather get close to a big juicy steak than a soup bone.

A BARTENDER: Sure, I like 'em big. I don't want to have to shake the sheets to find my woman.

A CONSTRUCTION WORKER: I want a lotta woman. I'm a big guy and a little bitty woman looks to me like a ... watch fob, and that ain't no woman.

A TEENAGER: Way down deep I dig 'em kinda fat and cuddly. But I don't date 'em because the guys would kid me. But when I get married, I am going to find me a chick with a little padding on her bones. They're cuter.

Ms. King admits that she also received negative answers, but says, "It would have been the same if I were asking them if they liked lavender sachet, asparagus, or golf. Some do and some don't."

Often, a man who likes his woman fat causes a problem for the woman who may be trying to lose weight or is worried about how she looks. She is confronted with a choice of pleasing herself or pleasing him. Greta says, "When I was my heaviest, I went with a guy who liked heavy women. I thought I looked absolutely horrible, and I felt disgusted with myself. When we talked about it, he said the fatter I was, the more he was turned on. I felt trapped. I knew that if I lost the weight he would lose interest."

## Do Women Really Like Fat Men?

Fat women do not necessarily have a reciprocal desire for fat men.

•

"If I went to all the trouble of losing a lot of weight, I wouldn't want to be with a fat man. When I'm fat, I know I can't be choosy, but when I'm thin, I think I can."

•

"I'm pretty liberal about it because I'm fat. A man would have to be really grossly overweight to be repulsive to me. I'm not turned off by men with a big gut. I'm turned off when the fat becomes bizarre looking."

•

Lewis and Olga have had a running quarrel throughout their twelve-year marriage. He insists that she be bone thin (which she is) and berates her whenever she gains a few pounds. He weighs close to 200 pounds. "Why can't Lewis lose some weight too? I stay thin for him. Why can't he make an effort for me?"

·

Karen, who is fat, likes fat men, but not because they are fat. "With a really skinny guy, sex is more of a threat. Physically, he's in control. It makes me feel inadequate. He knows something I don't know. Really thin people know something I don't know. It's frightening. Being around people who seem in control of themselves, I am less confident. Someone who is skinny, fit, or in touch with his body is better than I am because I don't feel I am any of those things. It's all right if I have something over the guy — if I have more power or money or if he's falling at my feet. Then I have control."

## Maneuvering for Position

Once in bed, most fat people don't have any trouble making love. Fat people are not usually maladjusted sexually. Their most common complaints are shortness of breath and fatigue. They have trouble with the logistics of sex, just moving around, and finding a position that will least reveal the big stomach, the lumps, or the hips.

·

Joshua, an obese man, cannot perform the way he would like to in bed. "I never know what to do with myself. I always feel so clumsy. My body gets in the way of everything. I'm always afraid I'm going to smother the woman. It's hard for me to rest on my elbows because of all that weight, and my stomach keeps getting in the way, preventing us from being really close. It's an obstacle, and there's no way to get around it. I always end up with the woman on top of me, even though it gives me less pleasure. It gets boring, always doing it in the same position, exactly the same way."

•

Patricia, a woman who generally likes heavy men ("There's more to hold on to"), said, "We were right in the middle, and all of a sudden he just collapsed and rolled off me. He was breathing very heavily, but it wasn't from passion. He was having trouble catching his breath. It was as if he'd been running. I was scared — I thought maybe he was having a heart attack — but after a few minutes he got himself together and we tried again. I was almost there when it happened again. This time I was angry. I didn't say anything though — how can you tell a fat man that he's too fat and he shouldn't be having sex unless he can follow through? Of course, I never saw him again."

## Lights Out

Mark, a gigolo who has been with more women than he can count, says of fat women, "The first thing is, they never get fully undressed with the lights on. They never walk around nude. They like the lights off during sex, and they clutch at the sheets a lot. They really think they're cool about not showing how lousy they feel about their bodies."

•

Jeannette refuses to get into certain positions. "I hate to be on top. I feel too exposed. I want to hide, and you can't hide from above."

•

Rosalyn's self-disgust is such that she feels she has no right to enjoy sex. "I can't relax. If a guy touches me, all I can think of are my bulges, and when we're in bed, I make sure that I'm all covered up. I have fantasies of abandonment, of being in all kinds of positions, doing everything I'd like to do, but I just don't dare."

•

Because of her fat, Donna remained a virgin until she was twenty-seven. She lives with a man now, but there are still problems. "If I eat something fattening, I have to wear my nightgown to bed. If I have sex with my boy friend, I feel somehow that I have to be passive. When I'm heavy, I don't want to be aggressive. I can't loosen up enough. I feel I have to hide my weight."

## It's Too Small

Raoul, who is in his early forties, is afflicted with a fear common to many men. "All my life I've felt that my penis was too small. Having five children hasn't helped — and I guess that's part of the reason I wanted a lot of children. My stomach is just too big. Even when I have an erection, I can't see my penis." Raoul's fear has played havoc with his sex life. He describes making love in a way that makes him appear sexually passive. He wants his wife to make the overture and needs strong indications from her that she will accept his lovemaking. They have developed a system of signals. "Did you brush your hair?" Raoul asks. If his wife says yes, it means that their lovemaking will proceed smoothly. Sometimes she says she is tired. Sometimes she nags him about his weight. Raoul gets back at her by eating junk food in front of her or by letting weeks pass without touching her.

## *Fear and Self-loathing*

Many obese people become confused and frightened when someone expresses strong sexual interest in them. Sex will strip their protective covering away. To counter the fear, they put themselves down, thus effectively putting themselves out of the picture. Their reaction is a variation on the old Groucho Marx line: "I wouldn't join a club that would have me as a member."

1. It must be my personality, my mind, my sense of humor that he (she) likes.

2. I must look very thin today, or else she (he) needs eyeglasses.

3. I have to keep this from going too far. I'd never want to be seen without my clothes.

4. If I don't like the way I look, how can anyone else?

5. If he (she) wants me, something must be wrong with him (her).

•

Nella met a man at a party. She wasn't too interested in him, but he pursued her. "He wrote me a letter saying he loved me because I was so fat and wonderful and big. I thought he was a sicko or something."

•

Ronnie says, "If somebody comes on to me, I always imagine he feels sorry for me. He's thinking, I'll do this out of duty to this poor fat person. I'll give her a thrill. Even if someone I love is turned on to me, I think I'm just getting sympathy sex."

## Feeling Like a Failure

When fat people look over their years of fat, of dieting and putting the weight back on, what stands out clearly is a history of failure. It's hard to face up to the number of times one has tried to lose weight and given up, slipped back into the old comforting but despised patterns. How much harder is it, then, to admit to another feeling of failure — sexual failure? The combination is devastating: the shame of having a fat body, the fear of appearing ugly to another person, and the fear of not being good in bed. Many fat people deal with this emotional clobbering by denying their sexuality.

•

Jason, who gained thirty pounds in three months, says, "Lately, I haven't had any sex at all. I've just kind of retreated into myself. I don't like dealing with all the entanglements and the romantic relationships. I always wind up feeling trapped. So I get into triangle situations where there is another man in the picture. To have sex with the woman would be a problem because she's going with someone, and I like her boy friend. Of course, there are a million women out there who are not tied up with my friends."

•

Melissa hides behind passivity and childlike behavior. She went from an all-girls' high school to a college that had just started to admit women. The ratio — fourteen men to one woman — overwhelmed her. As a protective device, she cultivated men as friends. "We put up boundaries and we categorized each other. No one stepped out of a pigeonhole. I felt safe. I got very close to one man who wasn't sexual with anyone. We discussed our fears. He said 'We're really close friends — any time you want to have sex, we'll try it.' We were like two little children; we made it sound so simple; we were so scared. There was a real sense that neither of us would hurt the other one."

•

A well-known Hollywood actress and singer who is 5 feet 3 inches and so round that she has to go on a starvation diet before each new film, says, "Fat men are like little boys. I was going with a notoriously obese rock musician. The closer we got to sex, the more kiddylike it became. Everything was baby talk, cutesy-poo, sweetheart — that sort of thing. The fat says, I'm not an adult; sex isn't serious."

•

Glen says, "After the initial sexual approach and before going to bed, I always talk about how horrible it is to love food. It's a Fat Confession, the way a married woman would tell you she has a husband. It's a way of making myself feel better about being fat and forestalling criticism of my body."

## Disembodied Brain

Sylvia, who has been obese all of her life, has managed to repress her sexual feelings and the sense of herself as a woman. She lives in sexual oblivion. She believes that her power is invested in her fat body and that she has remarkable intellectual ability. This combination of enhanced intelligence and power through weight is a common illusion among fat people. It is also a justification for staying fat.

"Ever since I was a child, I've pretended I didn't have a body and that people liked me because of my mind. I always knew I should try to lose weight. I've tried, but it never seemed important enough. I mean, I do all right."

## Safety First

Alice is secure in the knowledge that she is unattractive to men — but what about the one man in her life, Ed, her husband? After five years, their sex life is minimal, and they never discuss it. Alice rejects Ed's infrequent advances as often as she can, but once, the tables were turned — Alice wanted her husband. She had gone on a trip for a week. On the day she was to return, she called Ed and announced that she wanted to make love that night when she got back. After dinner, Ed busied himself with work he had brought home from the office while Alice sat and waited for him to make an advance. Finally, feeling totally rejected, she went to bed alone.

In reality, something entirely different had been going on. Alice had set up the situation by announcing her plan on the phone. Her control of the bed scene angered and intimidated Ed. She was pressuring him to perform at her command. The pressure guaranteed nothing but a fiasco for him, thereby eliminating the possibility of Alice's embarrassment and failure. Had she come home without making any grandiose announcements, Alice might have been confronted with the terrifying spectacle of Ed's desire and lust. Having arranged events, she could say that Ed's failure to show desire for her wasn't her fault; their failure to make love had nothing to do with her lack of desire or weight. She was safe.

## Thin Outside, Fat Inside

At one time or another, we've all heard someone say, "I may look thin, but inside I still feel fat." A letter from a formerly fat woman to Abigail van Buren, the columnist who gives advice as Dear Abby, illustrates the quandary:

DEAR ABBY,
I'm 29, married and mixed up. All my life I was a fat girl with a pretty face, but a good man fell in love with me and married me. Two years ago I took off 55 pounds. I love myself thin, but now I've got problems I never had before. Men started noticing me. I got involved with a man at work who gave me a line I was dumb enough to fall for. ("Divorce your husband and marry me.") Well, I asked my husband for a divorce — confessed everything, and then the other guy backed off. The rat! I felt like two cents. Thank God, my husband forgave me. Then I got involved with a married neighbor who had a reputation for fooling around. In the middle of that affair I started up another, with a salesman, younger than myself, who calls on our office. Abby, I never had these problems when I was fat. I don't want to be fat again, but the "new me" is so weak and trampy I can't stand to live with myself. Please help me. — THIN AND MIXED-UP

DEAR THIN: You apparently still think of yourself as the "fat girl no man would want." You need to keep proving to yourself that you're desirable. Get some counseling and become acquainted with the real you. I think you'll like her. (A real "tramp" wouldn't feel guilty.) — ABBY

## The Pre-rejection Syndrome

Saying no first is another approach to avoiding sex and its implications. This preventive method of operating is a risk-free guarantee that no one will ever say no to you. It protects you from the remotest possibility that someone might not want you. You may also cut yourself off from meeting new people and actually enjoying your life, but that is secondary to the terrible fear of rejection.

•

Bonnie, who is overweight, went to a disco with a thin girl friend. "I felt like a horse next to her." At the next table were two attractive men, one of whom asked her girl friend to dance. Then the second man asked Bonnie, who immediately assumed he was only being polite. As soon as she stood up he would realize his mistake. But she loves to dance. "I really got into it and forgot what I looked like. Luckily, it was dark, and I had a few drinks." After several dances, the men invited the women to another disco. Bonnie, who was having a good time, begged off. "I still felt he was being polite. He was probably wishing he had someone better looking to go out with. He was tall and well built. Why would he want to spend any money on me?"

Bonnie was afraid that the man might want to go to bed with her. She was also afraid that he might *not* want to go to bed with her. Either way, she couldn't win. Bonnie prefers fantasy to real life. She has created a drama in her mind and plays all the parts. The climax of her drama comes when the hero rejects her, and she becomes the suffering, spurned heroine — a role that frees her to eat.

## Fat in the Gay World

Sexual attitudes among gay people are not very different from those among heterosexual people. The flamboyant fringe gets publicity, leaving the impression that it is representative of the whole. Most gay men, like most straight men, tend to seek a beautiful partner. A slender, youthful body is of prime importance for sexual success.

·

Alex, who only recently "came out," has gained weight. "As soon as the reality of the gay scene hit me, I started eating enormously. It's so body oriented. Putting on a lot of weight keeps me away from the bars, which scare the hell out of me. If I'm fat, I can tell myself I'm not attractive enough to meet anybody, so I stay home and don't bother."

·

Luke too gained weight out of fear. "I've been living with a guy for about four years. Three years ago, I began to realize that my lover was not monogamous. I was going to have to see other people too. But I was freaked out by the whole gay scene. I gained a lot of weight. I'm either going to have to lose it or spend a lot of time alone."

·

Ken has had only one lover in his life. After two years he is getting restless but is afraid to risk rejection. "I went to a couple of gay bars just to see what they were like. I didn't think anyone would want to pick me up. I saw some really attractive guys, and I wanted to ask them to dance, but I was sure they wouldn't want to dance with me. They were all slender. I'm scared for emotional reasons, not only because I'm heavy."

·

Most gay women, like most heterosexual women, stress emotional intimacy more than good looks. They seek closeness. Although looks are an important part of any sexual attraction, gay women seem largely able to accept each other for who they are as women and for the love and feelings they give each other. Many gay women have discarded male values that have been imposed on *all* women — in particular, that women have to be attractive in order to please men.

·

"At one time you had to get a man and you had to get married," Margie said. "You married to get out of the house, and you hoped it would be different than it was at home. You thought that maybe marriage would make men seem more attractive and interesting. That's all changed now. There's no reason to conform to male ideas of what you should like and be."

·

Iris looks for personality. However, she does discriminate between fatness and obesity. "When I meet a woman, my first reaction is to her soul. But if she is obese — even if I like her face — I couldn't get to her soul. Apart from that, it's the emotional thing that turns me on. If ten naked women walked across this floor and you asked me to pick one, I couldn't. Physical appearance does very little for me. I would probably pick the ugliest body if she had the nicest personality."

## Dehumanized

Fat women generally feel deeply offended by society's expectation that first and foremost they must be attractive sexually, that their main purpose in life is to be a sex object. They consider their real value as human beings to encompass more than just the physical. By emphasizing the physical and the sexual, they feel, society turns them into something less than human. Women feel it's the whole person that counts. It angers them when they think men want them only for their bodies. Becoming fat and unattractive is their way of protecting themselves against being a sex object.

.

Denise believes the old dumb-blonde stereotype about women — that if you're beautiful you can't also be intelligent. "It's very dangerous, losing weight. All of a sudden you're a pretty woman, you're a body. And that's what men are interested in. Then you have to ask yourself, 'Well, don't I have more to give? Don't I have a mind too?' So you try to make yourself ugly to relieve the anxiety."

.

Laura has discovered that men aren't interested in her unless she's thin. "When I used to sleep with a lot of men, I was the thinnest I ever was. I was so thrilled with being thin that I wanted to use my body — I *wanted* to be an object at that point. It was that or nothing. I never thought I was attractive. It's a double bind. They don't care about *you,* just if you're fat or thin. And my response is, the hell with you; I'm going to eat and if you don't love me don't touch me."

.

Amy says, "I lost a lot of weight, and I started going to singles bars and being with a lot of men and really loving it — and then it started to scare me. I started gaining weight. I was using the sex for myself, proving to myself that I could be attractive — but now, I don't want only that. I know I'm attractive. I had to gain the weight back and reverse myself so men wouldn't want me only for my body."

## Ostrich

It is important to Louise's self-image that she be able to go to a party and be found attractive by a man. Louise is often successful, but one thing puzzles her — the men she takes home with her almost never ask her out to lunch or dinner or anyplace else public. Often they don't even call her back, even though, according to Louise, the lovemaking works out well. Louise has the faculty of being able to ignore her weight. She just pretends it isn't there. She is like an ostrich, sticking her head in the sand to avoid facing reality. "I don't think I'm fat. I think I look good. I'm well proportioned, and I don't see myself as less attractive than other women. But I don't understand why, when I get a guy to come home with me, I don't feel better about myself when he leaves." Louise is aware that she won't find a boy friend if she keeps having casual sex, but casual sex makes her feel attractive. It has become a quick fix, like food. Without it, she would have to face the truth about her weight.

## Food as a Substitute for Sex

Food and sex are both very sensual, and many people use one when they don't have the other. If you don't have someone to make you feel satisfied and fulfilled, eating will do it for you. Food is love. But there is another twist to the equation. Some obsessive overeaters use food even when they have enough sex.

•

Arthur says, "When I met Jill I really started gaining weight again. She's very good in bed. She really satisfies me. But

I still overeat. When there isn't a woman in my life, I tell myself it's because I'm fat, and I figure I'd better lose some weight. When I have someone, I forget the other stuff and feel happy and satisfied. What is it about? What am I doing?" Arthur uses any reason he can find to eat. He eats when he feels bad, and he eats when he feels good. Addicts use drugs the same way. Arthur is a foodaholic.

•

Many people, whether they are fat or thin, prevent themselves from just enjoying the sheer physical pleasure of lovemaking. They bring self-consciousness, feelings of inadequacy, fear of intimacy, and other irrelevant issues into bed, where such problems don't belong. They create their own sexual problems. If your sex life is not all that you would like it to be, you can always put the blame on your fat. The fat is an excuse for sexual failure, and sexual failure is a paradigm for all the failures in your life. Everything wrong can be blamed on your fat. It is painful to feel undesirable in a world where everyone else seems to be desirable, but the fat and the pain are lesser evils than the alternative: doing something about your problems, becoming responsible for yourself.

# 9

# Taking It Off
# and Keeping It Off:
# The Secret Ingredient

*"O! that this too too solid flesh would melt,*
*Thaw and resolve itself into a dew . . ."*

HAVE YOU EVER met an old friend unexpectedly, someone you haven't seen in a long time, and almost not recog-
nized her? The change is striking. She's lost all flab and
pulled herself together. She looks like a brand-new person.
You feel a surge of envy — and a burning curiosity. How
did she do it?

At a meeting of professional people, I ran into a therapist I had not seen for several years. I remembered her as
having elephantine proportions, a tall woman whose width
matched her height. I was astonished at the changes in the
way she looked. She now carried herself with grace and
walked purposefully, slouch and waddle gone. There was
a new look about her: more confident, much more attractive, even to the clothes she was wearing. She looked thin
even though she wasn't.

I complimented her on the change, and asked her how

she had done it. She said she had lost eighty pounds and had forty more to go. She spoke of going to a doctor and dieting, and I interrupted her. What I really wanted to know, I explained, was how she had made the decision to lose weight and how she had managed to stay with it. I hoped to hear a formula of some kind, a recitation of easy steps to taking action, or a dramatic episode in her life that had changed everything. Even a tale of agonizing psycho-analytic sessions that had broken through to some deep-rooted problem and freed her to lose weight. Her answer was simple. "I don't know. I just did it."

I have asked the same question of almost everyone I know who once was fat. What compelled them to lose weight? Where did they get the determination to stick to their guns? What is the secret? To the great chagrin of fat people, physicians, psychiatrists, and therapists, the answer is always the same: "I don't know. One day I just decided to do it."

## The Secret Ingredient

You know all the problems about yourself — all the neurotic longings that keep you fat. You know you're a baby needing to be fed. You feel deprived without your consolation food; if you don't eat as much as you think you want you're dissatisfied, empty inside. Food binds up the wounds that the world inflicts on you; it protects you from grappling with fears and problems you can't face. Eating is something to hide behind, a barrier between you and the threat of intimacy with others.

You've tried all the diets, everything from Atkins to

Weight Watchers to Scarsdale, and you gained the pounds back. You've starved and fasted. Nothing has worked for you. You're in despair, doomed to be forever fat, forever ugly, forever sitting on the sidelines of life. Everyone is familiar with the cliché: Within every fat person there is a thin person trying to get out. Who sentenced you to this prison?

Somewhere inside, being fat was more important to you than anything else in the world. Whatever you needed, whatever it was you got from being fat, far outweighed the benefits of being thin. When that equation shifts in your head, you will be able to lose weight. When you want something more than you want to be fat, and when getting it requires that you lose weight, you will lose weight. When losing weight is its own reward, you will lose weight.

The secret ingredient is, of course, *you*. You are the reason why you haven't lost weight, and you are the reason why you will lose weight. Your desire, your will, your determination are decisive. That desire is often combined with a compelling passion or a complex network of reasons that work together for you. It may be conscious or unconscious.

Your secret ingredient could be an overriding need to control your life. It could be hidden anger, rage, the imperative urge to get back at your family for what they did to you as a child. It could be the status of a job promotion, or sheer economic necessity. The desire for a lover, the need for independence. It could be a yearning to look attractive, an image of yourself as lean and competent, as a superior tennis player, as a man about town or a woman of mystery. Or wanting to be "normal," just like everyone else. It could be such a deep self-loathing, such an overwhelming need to change your life, that starving would be preferable to your current situation. Whatever your secret ingredient is, it touches your inner core; it is entwined with your deepest longings.

The secret ingredient acts as a trigger. For some people there is no discernible trigger, no concrete desire to make them lose weight. They just do it. It just seems to happen, and they can't explain it. For others, an insignificant incident is enough to set them off. For Bob, sugar lost its savor, and the self-motivation gear clicked into place. He went along with his feeling. He cut down on sweets and extended the ban to starches. He lost weight, and the result was so felicitous that he never gained it back.

The trigger, conscious or not, is part of your psychological makeup. It is different for each person. No one can find your secret ingredient for you. That is your responsibility.

Losing weight won't necessarily be physically healthy or esthetically pleasant. I think of Kate, who said, "I'd rather be dead than fat," and went to a Dr. Feelgood for pills and injections. Kate is self-destructive: she eats junk food, gives in to her pizza cravings, and drinks too much at parties — but she keeps the weight off.

·

Charlotte couldn't stop eating but decided she wanted a man more than she wanted the food she loved. She started carrying chicken legs around with her. "Broiled chicken legs aren't fattening," she said, somewhat embarrassed by her behavior. When other people in the office are having a Danish and coffee at 10:30 in the morning, Charlotte has a chicken leg. Between coffee breaks and lunch, ashamed to let everyone see how often she eats, she goes to the ladies' room to get her chicken-leg fix. "Hiding in a stall is not exactly an elegant way to eat," she concedes, "but it's a lot better than eating cake."

.

Kate and Charlotte have made their priorities.

## Making Positive Decisions

The following stories are of people who gained control over their fat problem and chose not to be fat. They stopped making excuses for themselves. They unlocked their prison doors. Each did it according to his or her own lights. In one way or another, each found his or her own secret ingredient.

.

Hal had always set himself discouraging goals of large numbers of pounds to lose and given up in despair well short of achieving them. One day he decided that numbers were madness. He has taken command of the scale. "I've forgotten about pounds. I'm going to lose enough weight so that when I look in the mirror I can say I like what I see."

.

Cheryl too has made her peace with numbers. The scale no longer rules her life. She thinks about losing two or three pounds at a time — a series of little goals that are manageable. She weighs herself once a week, no more, and if she has lost only one pound in a particular week, that's all right too.

.

Dennis has come to terms with his binges. He diets rigorously — except when he goes on a binge. In the past he would give up his diet after each binge, using the binge as an excuse for a relapse. Now he realizes that if he loses five pounds on his diet and gains back three from a binge, he has lost two pounds. A two-pound weight loss is a reason to rejoice.

•

Peggy has stopped spending a lot of money in the grocery store. "I live alone, and there's no reason to be tempted by a full refrigerator. Mostly, I eat eggs and tuna fish. I want to look good, so I spend food money on clothes."

•

Polly's family helped her to lose weight once they realized she was serious. They agreed to eliminate sugar and desserts at home, and they saw to it that Polly ate half-portions during family meals.

•

Jean, a divorced thirty-four-year-old mother of two children, works and studies for her bachelor's degree two nights a week. All her life Jean was accustomed to living well. Now she receives neither alimony nor child support and is in desperate financial straits. She needs her degree to qualify for a better-paying job. She is so busy and so focused on her economic goals that she forgets about food. "I still long for certain kinds of foods, but other things are more important."

•

Keith discovered he was on the wrong kind of diet. "I tried to eat diet foods and salads. I stayed away from red meat. But I was raised to believe that red meat is necessary for me. When I'm not eating it, I'm constantly hungry. I can never get enough of other foods to make up for that lack.

Nothing else fills me up. I realized that if I had one hamburger or steak, I wouldn't be hungry. I've lost weight since then. I'm convinced that a lot of fat people are starving because of their crazy ideas of what the 'right' diet foods should be."

.

Linda stays away from health foods. They don't satisfy her, and she ends up eating twice as much. "Salads and vegetables are a waste of time. The last time I went to a health-food place, I had a raw vegetable salad and fruit salad, but I was the only person who ate bread. Afterward, I was starving for something real. I found a little bakery and had something I actually like — apple pie. Then I wasn't hungry for hours."

.

Stanley finally forgave his parents for the terrible time they gave him as a child. His huge load of guilt and anger dropped away, releasing him from the need to overeat.

.

Amy found her motivation in reverse revenge. "I lost fifty pounds after breaking a long relationship. I thought, well, screw you. Now that you don't want me anymore, I'm going to show you. I'm going to be gorgeous."

.

Dolores has lost large quantities of weight twice in her life, each time stimulated by an important event. "I lost sixty pounds after I broke up with Jack. I'm not sure what made me go through with it. Probably being alone. I saw that I had to do it to meet someone else. The second time was after I moved away from home into my own apartment. Both times were a big change in my life — having to look after myself."

## Taking Charge

Helen got fed up with her life. Her teaching job had turned sour; she was thirty-five, weighed 247 pounds, and half her life was over. She decided to take control, to direct her life instead of going along with events passively. Helen quit her job and went to a spa for a week to begin her new program on the right foot. "I've changed my eating habits. I'm not feeding my problems anymore. My brother got me a food processor for Valentine's Day. I use it to shred carrots for carrot salad. His present was a nice surprise. He used to give me candy. It's hard for me to pass certain bakeries, certain restaurants, but my reward is watching that scale go down. I get on the scale twice a day, sometimes more. I have no reason to be afraid anymore. A guy walked out on me, but I didn't eat over it."

·

For Chuck, 6 feet 2 inches and 240 pounds, the spur was ridicule. "My family started calling me Hulk. I was really hurt. I didn't see myself as being obese. When I wanted a beer, my brother would say, 'Yeah, I'll get you a beer, Hulk.' My sister painted a Christmas gift plate for me that said, 'Merry Christmas to the Hulk.' It was like a slap in the face. They made me feel like a stupid clod. At first I thought I would overeat to get back at them, but I realized I'd only get fatter. I started to fight back. Every time I reached for a bag of potato chips I stopped myself by saying *Hulk*. I hated being fat. When I went to a health club and the instructor asked, 'When did you start bulkin' up?' that was my second knock on the head.

"I started by fasting the first two days. The third day I

had some fruit. Then I ate one meal a day, no breakfast. Instead of potato chips, an apple; instead of Coke, plain soda. It was agony. Now I eat a lot of vegetables, fish, chicken. I take vitamins. I eat whole-wheat bread. I was a Wonder Bread child. I still like it, but I don't go near it. I have to be conscious of what I'm eating all the time. At breakfast, I have to fight not to have pancakes and syrup. If I even start, I don't like myself, and I don't feel healthy. I'm down to 165. Now my problem is excess skin. Exercise helps. Since I've been roller-skating, I lost an inch and a half on my thighs. It felt so good to get my first pair of designer jeans. Everyone asks me how I did it. When I tell them, they all say, 'Oh, I could never do that.' They could if they put their minds to it. They don't want to."

•

Buffy got disgusted. Knocking about the world a bit after school and stranded in Malaysia, Buffy lived as the poor did, on a diet consisting mainly of rice. She lost thirty-five pounds. "When I came home, I realized how little food I needed to survive. It made me ill to watch people gorging themselves. I made a decision not to eat more than my body needed. I've become incapable of overeating. I know when to stop. Instead of the pleasure of half a gallon of ice cream, I have the pleasure of slim legs."

•

Joe needed a support system, a surrogate family to give him the love and care he lacked as a child. "Living in San Francisco with a girl, I really wanted to break away. During that time, my body just blew up. I put on fifty pounds in one year. I didn't even notice it. The weight just sort of attached itself to me. One day, suddenly, there I was — fat.

"Single again, I was free and loose, but I was a fat guy.

I couldn't resign myself to being fat. I still thought of myself as I used to be. It was rough because I had been kind of a flirty guy, a happy-go-lucky person. There were times when I thought, 'Wow, she's a doll, but the chick wouldn't look twice at me.' Suddenly the choice wasn't mine anymore. Loneliness was the biggest thing, the long periods of not seeing anybody, or waking up with somebody I'd just picked up in a bar and didn't ever want to see again. The loneliness was the same as when I'd been a fat boy. I think the only satisfaction I got when I was growing up was a good meal.

"I didn't know how to lose weight. I was ignorant of what makes you fat and what doesn't. After a year of being fat, I tried to diet. I would do something ridiculously Spartan like starve myself, then put the weight back on again. I put it back on because there was no satisfaction.

"Now I've found some new friends. They were on the Stillman diet, and we supported each other, like a family. I've taken off forty pounds and would like to lose another twenty. No more fat Joe. It started as a New Year's resolution. I thought, O.K., I've tried everything, and this time I'm not going to be hard on myself. If there was a day I could go without eating, I'd go without eating. If not, not. I'm pulling myself together. I found a new job. Losing weight isn't an isolated thing; it's part of the program."

•

Lucy, who is twenty-six years old and 5 feet 1 inch, went from 168 to 123 pounds. She became aware of herself as a woman. "When I was growing up, I didn't see many women who took care of themselves. We lived in a neighborhood where women wore housedresses and no makeup and got fat. My mother was like that. I sort of blame her for my weight problem. I didn't have any sense of her as a woman.

"My present boss is a chic, well-groomed, slender woman who has two grown daughters. I can't help thinking she must have been a lousy mother. I know how ridiculous that sounds, but the mother image to me is a shlep — overweight, aproned, always cooking. My mother didn't work.

"I lost weight because I wanted something from all the people in group therapy, but especially from Mark. I have fantasies about him. When he said he didn't like me because I was fat, I really sat up and took notice. It was a challenge. I started looking at what I was eating. I don't like diets. I have an orange for breakfast. For lunch, yogurt or a little container of cottage cheese with lettuce and tomato. Very small portions. For dinner, a piece of broiled fish or chicken, or sometimes a big salad with some tuna fish in it. I don't seem to have a need for binges, even though I still have an oral fixation. Whenever I get nervous, I drink a cup of herb tea or a glass of water, or I chew gum.

"I know this has to be my lifestyle, and I never allow myself to get into a funk about being denied goodies. When I go out, I eat bread and even dessert, but the next day I take care of it. I've had so much anger and misery in my life, hated my body, hated myself — this is one part of my life now where I am treating myself well.

"Even now that I've lost weight, I still feel fat. At work when I go into the bathroom to put on makeup with the other women, I'm ashamed. I think they think, 'Who is she kidding?' I'm afraid people will laugh at me for trying to be like a woman. I spent so many years in T-shirts and paint-stained dungarees. I still feel unfeminine and sexless. Now that I feel good about myself, I'm going to get some other things together — clothes and makeup. I'm going to take care of myself. When I was fat, it didn't matter. I have an appointment tomorrow to have a manicure, the first in my whole life. I'm trying to get used to feeling like a woman instead of the blob I used to be. I don't want to be a fat person anymore."

•

Harriet wanted to escape from her family to become someone else entirely, a person living a life different from anything she had known. "I was a fat child. I hated myself, hated the way I looked. I was different from other children, and I didn't know how to get along with them. I never belonged. I couldn't relax and play with them and be part of the group. I stood outside and watched myself, how I looked, how I acted. And I envied all the other little girls their skinny bodies and the way they laughed so easily.

"My mother and grandmother took care of me. They were old-fashioned women who looked after their families and their houses and didn't want to do anything else. All their energy went into me, an only child. They dressed me, fed me, bathed me. I felt they were like vultures, picking at me. I felt like a lump, a thing, not a person. I didn't know how to do anything.

"They believed that children should be plump. *Fat* meant 'health' to them. My mother spoon-fed me until I was six years old. There was always plenty of good, solid food. We had potatoes with almost every meal. The food I was given was 'good for me.' The idea of pleasure did not enter into eating. You ate because you would die if you didn't.

"I was considered a picky eater, but I think it was more that I didn't like the same foods my mother did. She liked sour cream and refused to believe that I didn't. Every day at lunch she would try to feed me sour cream out of the container, and I would gag on it and not swallow it, just sit with it in my mouth until finally I spit it out. Every day she tried again. She was five feet tall and weighed 145 pounds, and I found her disgusting to look at. She bulged everywhere. I didn't like her to touch me.

"Dinners were arguments. Why didn't I finish my steak? Why hadn't I touched my vegetables? My mother jumped up and down waiting on everyone, running back and forth from the kitchen to clear the table, like a servant. There was no conversation. I couldn't wait to leave the table. My father never said much. Occasionally he told my mother to leave me alone. He couldn't stand fights. After a day at the office, he wanted peace. I was drawn to him. He was a man of the world, above all this petty squabbling. He didn't pick at me.

"When I was twelve, I went to summer camp. I discovered that I was coordinated. I was good at sports. For the first time in my life, I belonged. I was chosen to be on the basketball, volleyball, and softball teams; I was sought after. People actually liked me. The world opened up. I saw other girls who looked the way I wanted to look and said clever things that I wanted to say. I copied them, taking bits and pieces from each one. Slowly the idea grew in my head of the person I wanted to be.

"I wasn't sure how to lose weight. I thought people were either naturally fat or naturally thin, born that way and stuck with it for the rest of their lives. Everyone I knew ate too much, including the thin people. They just never gained weight. When food packages arrived from home, the thin campers stuffed themselves too.

"Back in the city, the vision of that other person I wanted

to be stayed with me. Each year it got stronger, and the older I got, the more possible it became. When I left home I would be that person and have an exciting life. Whatever happened, I would never in any way be like my mother. Above all, I would not be a fat mindless woman who turned herself inside out for everyone else and got no thanks for it.

"It took six years, but gradually the vision overwhelmed the food. I stopped eating foods that were good for me — milk, orange juice, cheese, potatoes, even fruit and vegetables. I stuck to foods I liked, foods that satisfied me and made me feel good: bread and meat, black coffee, an occasional dessert. The scenes at the dinner table grew worse, but I was older now; I didn't care as much. By the time I left home for college, I was ready to be the person I had invented. I weighed 108 pounds. I'm forty now, and I've never gained back more than two pounds of it."

## Taking Responsibility

Once you make the decision to lose weight and come to terms with the sacrifice required, the next step is maintenance — figuring out which foods work for you and how much of them you can eat. The tricks you use to help yourself have to be part of your life, not imposed on you from outside. They have to be integrated with your likes and dislikes and synchronized with the pattern of your days. It doesn't do to work out a no-lunch diet when your dinner hour is 8 P.M. Somewhere between 8 A.M. and 8 P.M. you'll fill up on junk and ruin your diet program.

·

Sonny had to accommodate her solo eating habits to those of her lover when he moved in with her. "Being alone made the difference in losing a lot of weight. I could control what I ate. I didn't have to go to a bar and resist a beer or go to a restaurant and deal with heavy sauces. When I fell in love, it got very difficult. When someone is there and he loves you the way you are, what do you have to diet for? You think, 'Why am I being silly? Let's have a few drinks.' Bruce really liked to eat too. We both loved to cook and try new restaurants. That was a large part of our affair. But I had to maintain something, some kind of diet. I ate everything, but I ate small amounts. I drank half my drink and nibbled at the edges of scalloped potatoes. When Bruce wasn't around, I didn't eat meals."

·

Mai Ling satisfies her gluttonous appetite with her own special diet. "After two months of strenuous dieting, it became clear that the only way I could continue was by cheating. Every diet I know says you can never cheat. You're going to cheat on a diet, and you're going to gain the weight back unless you cheat very carefully. I started cheating on Sundays. I'd have pancakes, cheeseburgers, french fries, chocolate shakes — and then go right back on the diet. I lost over 100 pounds that way. After a few years, I started cheating three times a week. Days of cheating are days of happiness. I hardly eat anything on the days I don't cheat. It's a very flexible plan. I'm cheating today, but if I were going to a party tomorrow I wouldn't eat today."

·

Bonnie is a former bulimarexic. "I noticed that I was getting little breakages in the veins of my face from the pressure on my head from forced vomiting. I'm no longer hysterical about my size or about losing weight. I don't plan to let my weight get so bad that I get hysterical. I don't want to be that crazy. I don't throw up anymore. It seemed like a childish way out of my predicament. It was wholly self-destructive.

"I think about throwing up when I'm depressed and want pizza or want to gorge myself. But I found a way around it. I order pizza, eat two slices, and freeze the rest. I can have a little pizza for the rest of the week. It's a very conscious act. I have a discussion with myself. If I didn't think it through, I would probably just go ahead and eat the whole platter. There are tricks I use. I don't bring the whole pizza to where I'm eating. I warm it in the kitchen, divide it into two or three dinners, and freeze it. I go into another room with what I decide to eat that night. Also, I always start small. I start with two slices. I know that after two slices I'll be full. If I really want another slice, I can go back to the kitchen and unfreeze it. That makes me very aware that I'm overeating."

•

Ruth designed her own weight-loss program virtually from scratch. "You have to come to terms with food — eating what you need to eat — and keep everything in small amounts not to drive yourself crazy. You have to know what kinds of foods satisfy you and what kinds don't. You say, now is the time to lose weight and you do it. I kept going off my diet, but I was still very careful. It took me about seven months to lose twenty-eight pounds. I weighed myself two or three times a day. I still do. You step on the scale in the morning to see how much leeway you've got. My normal weight is 125 pounds. If the scale says 123, I have a good time that day — but not a completely, utterly good time. I don't really trust the scale because the next day I could get on it and weigh 127. But I trust the scale far enough to give me a little freedom. If it says 127 I'm careful that day or for two days, until it says 125 again.

"I'm an eater. I really like food. I really like the sensuousness of it, the texture, the chewing part, the taste, the cooking; I like everything about it. I've learned there are foods I really like and foods that are just a habit. So I tried to think of ways to eliminate the foods that were just a habit. I like the crunchy parts of french bread, so I just eat the outsides. I like textures. I like baked potato skins; the potato I can live without. I don't use oil in salad dressings. I get a very good vinegar and mix it with my favorite mustard. I have skimmed milk in my cappuccino. For breakfast I eat toast and eggs. Cereal and milk I have no use for.

"I like the texture of tuna fish salad but not oil and mayonnaise. You can eat tuna with yogurt, or you can take low-fat cottage cheese and blend it with lemon juice. This turns into something that tastes exactly like sour cream, which is cleaner tasting than mayonnaise. I use fresh dill and basil and herbs like that and make dressing just as soupy as I like it. It all depends on how you want food to look on your plate and how you want it to look on your fork and how you want it to feel in your mouth.

"There are ways to get around using butter. I use a lot of broth for flavor and very little oil. You sauté with chicken broth and a little bit of fat. You put a teeny little bit of fat on the bottom of the pan to dry-brown meat. I have a soapstone grill — pioneers used it for pancakes — that doesn't ever need oil. It gets very very hot and heats evenly.

"When I get an urge for something to eat, I analyze it. What do I want? Chocolate? How do I want the chocolate?

I really think about food so that when I eat it I know I'm getting what I want and I don't have the same urge two minutes later because it wasn't really what I wanted. Your body talks to you if you stop long enough to listen. The other day I thought I wanted some ice cream, and I ate some. Then I realized I would have preferred a bowl of strawberries with yogurt and honey. I think it was because I'm programmed to want ice cream when it's hot. When the ice cream was in my stomach I was disappointed in it. I still want that extra cream puff, but I can't go through another diet like the last one. I'm always consciously saying no. I push the plate away. It probably will be like that for the rest of my life."

•

The people whose stories you have just read count themselves among the formerly fat. For all you know, half the thin people you see on the street were once fat. They are free of the excess baggage they have been carrying around for most of their lives. You too can be one of them.

Formerly fat people know they must remain vigilant. Their old desires and habits still lurk under the surface. They have struggled through all phases of dieting and never want to return to the shame, the isolation, the self-hatred. They will never be fat again. When they do put on a few pounds, they will lose the weight immediately, catching themselves in time to prevent reliving old fat patterns.

Every one of us has the ability to make the same decision — to lose weight and to stay thin. Anyone who manages to lose weight *wants* to be thin, wants to badly enough to surmount the difficulties of becoming thin.

You alone have the power to change your body. You don't have to be fat. The choice to be thin is yours.